Prostate cancer is the most common form of cancer diagnosed in American men. After deaths due to lung cancer, prostate cancer is the next leading cause of death among men in the United States. Each year 334,500 men in America are diagnosed with new cases of prostate cancer; *more than **40,000 will die of it!***

Since 1991, incidences of prostate cancer have increased by 90%. This startling figure is partially due to the aging of the American population and a growing awareness of the disease and the widespread screening programs now in place. One in every ten men will develop clinically significant prostate cancer. It will be the cause of death to **3%** of the American male population.

This book will tell **everything** you need to know to detect prostate cancer before it worsens. Hopefully, it will be instrumental to your getting a yearly exam that will enable you to **prevent and cure** this dreadful disease.

Read it! It could save your life!

PROSTATE CANCER

Detection and Cure

by

A.M. Durrani, M.D., F.R.C.S.

Swan Publishing
Texas ❖ California ❖ New York

Author: Dr. A.M. Durrani
Editors: Pete Billac and Joseph DeJongh
Cover Design: Cliff Evans, Shelby Berry and Cindy Coker
Cover Coordination: Warren Waters
Layout Design: Sharon Davis

Prostate Cancer: Detection and Cure, is available in quantity discounts through: SWAN Publishing, 126 Live Oak, Alvin, TX 77511.
(281) 388-2547 or Fax (281) 585-3738.

Printed in the United States of America.

The ideas, procedures, and suggestions in this book are not intended as a substitute for the medical advice of a trained health professional. All matters regarding your health require medical supervision. Consult your physician before adopting the suggestions in this book, as well as any condition that may require diagnosis or medical attention. The author and publisher disclaim any liability arising directly or indirectly from the use of techniques in this book.

DEDICATION

To Najma, my wife, and to Sikandar and Omar my sons, for the encouragement they have given me and for their understanding. My profession and my writing have taken time away from them, but they know I love them dearly.

ACKNOWLEDGMENT

I am very fortunate to find several people to help me in the preparation of this book. I am especially indebted to my publisher, Pete Billac, for the invaluable editing and general supervision. His wife, Sharon, has been very kind to give a creative layout design to the book.

I am also grateful to Dr. John Libertino for his encouragement and the well-written foreword and to Dr. Carl Chan for his time in reviewing the chapter on radiation.

INTRODUCTION

I am a physician, a urologist, and my speciality is dealing with impotence and prostate cancer besides general urology. I also perform vasectomies and reversals. This book is written for all who want to know about the **detection** and **cure** of prostate cancer and to give hope to those who are diagnosed with the dreaded disease. I will do my utmost to simplify everything but I will also go into more detail for those who want to know more.

The mortality rate from prostate cancer is twice as high in **African-American** men as in Caucasian-American men. Also, the Incidence of significant prostate cancer in African Americans is usually larger at the time of *diagnosis,* and carries a poorer *prognosis*.

Prostate cancer has a strong familial tendency; history of prostate cancer in a father or a brother *doubles* the risk of developing this cancer. The risk increases **five fold** when more than one close member of the family has it. The exact reason for this association is unknown. It may be due to common dietary or environmental factors or it may have a genetic component.

Prostate cancer becomes increasingly more common with **advancing age**; it is commonly found in men over 65. Less than 1% are found in under 50. Often these tumors are very small and non-aggressive, causing no effects on health.

Diet plays a very important role in the development and progression of certain cancers. Dietary factors are implicated in about 50% of all cancers, and a diet with high fat content has been associated with increased risk of having this disease. A high-fat diet has been correlated with increased production of testosterone and clinical studies have shown that administration of testosterone causes prostate cancer in laboratory animals.

Mortality from prostate cancer is low in countries where diet is low in fat. In such places like Japan, where their diet has **four times less fat** than the western diet, Japanese men have the lowest incidence of the cancer. Low-fat diet may also substantially reduce the risk of developing prostate cancer. Black American men are at a much higher risk than those living in Africa, since their diet is also lower in fat.

There are several questions men want answered right now and I will do my best to answer them all, the simplest and easiest way. As a physician, it is logical—even normal—for me to tell more than you might care to know. I'll be specific and as much to the point as I am able, but please, indulge me. The more you know, the easier it is to *prevent* prostate cancer, the easier it is to **detect it early**, and the easier it is to treat and cure.

Dr. A. M. Durrani

TABLE OF CONTENTS

FOREWORD

The American Cancer Society estimates that 317,000 men will be diagnosed with prostate cancer in 1996, compared with 184,000 women with breast cancer. It is also anticipated that approximately 41,000 men will die of metastastic prostate cancer this year. From these statistics we can see that prostate cancer is a major medical condition that warrants our attention.

The public at large requires contemporary information to understand this disease and the various treatment options available. With this in mind, Dr. Durrani wrote this book, written in simple language so that non-physicians can understand the subject. Hopefully, this will help patients and their families (in conjunction with physicians) to decide in the treatment of prostate cancer.

This fine book includes chapters that deal with incidence, signs and symptoms, diagnosis, pathology and treatment options such as surgery, radiation therapy, cryosurgery, chemotherapy and hormonal treatment. Dr. Durrani wrote it from the perspective of a practicing urologist with over 20 years of experience.

On a personal level, I am very proud of Dr. Durrani, one of my former students. He has made a very valuable contribution not only to the specialty of urology, but to the patients and their families who are interested in finding out more about this dreaded disease. *Prostate Cancer:*

Detection and Cure is a well-written, much needed, complete guide of a disease which plagues men throughout the world in ever increasing numbers.

John A. Libertino, M.D.

Chairman, Department of Urology
Chairman, Division of Surgery
Lahey Hitchcock Medical Center
Burlington, MA

Assistant Clinical Professor of Surgery
Harvard Medical School
Boston, MA

Part 1

The Prostate

To better understand prostate cancer, let's begin with where the prostate is. The base of the prostate lies under the urinary bladder. The *urethra* tube (through which urine is eliminated) passes through the middle of the prostate from its base above to the apex below.

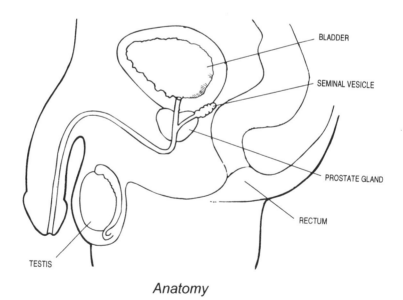

Anatomy

It is chestnut-shaped and about 20 grams (approx. ¾ of an ounce) in weight in an adult male. After age 50 it starts to grow larger.

The **function of the prostate** is as an accessory **male sex organ** composed of several small glands which secrete prostatic fluid during ejaculation. The prostatic fluid forms 80% of the seminal fluid which helps in the transport and survival of sperm.

Nerves responsible for erection of the penis lie behind the prostate, and along with the blood vessels, form a neurovascular bundle. The prostate is important during the reproductive life of an individual. In later life, it serves no useful function and instead becomes the most common site of disease in man.

DETECTING PROSTATE CANCER

Prostrate cancer is being detected more than ever because men are becoming increasingly aware of the disease and undergo yearly physical exams. I cannot emphasize enough, the necessity of a yearly exam. It is a way of detecting prostate cancer before it worsens. In the past several years, **random** screening programs are being conducted around the country on healthy men where evidence of prostate cancer shows up.

The early stages of prostate cancer are often *without* symptoms; 45% of the patients discovered to have this cancer from screening *had no symptoms.* When symptoms do appear, they are often difficult to distinguish from those stemming from a benign enlargement of the prostate, where the symptoms usually appear slowly and take a long time to develop. The symptoms of prostate cancer intensify more quickly.

IF ANY OF THESE SYMPTOMS APPEAR, SEE YOUR PHYSICIAN

✔If you have the urge to urinate **frequently** and a need to wake up at night to do so, these are signs of an irritation of the prostate. Make an appointment with your physician!

✔If you have a **leakage** of urine, it is caused by an obstruction of the bladder outlet caused by an enlarged prostate which in turn causes the urine to overflow from a constantly full bladder.

✔If there is a **hesitancy**, where urination does not start immediately when desired or starts after some delay, be aware that there might be a problem. This occurs more often in the mornings when the bladder is too full to force the urine through the resistance of an enlarged prostate. Call your doctor!

✔If you have the **inability** to urinate, this is due to a blockage of the urine outlet from the bladder. Retention occurs more commonly in benign enlargement of the prostate. Still, make that call!

✔If you should see occasional **blood** (Hematuria) in the urine, there is a problem. Don't hesitate! Make that appointment with your physician.

Yes, early detection can save your life! Starting at age 50, every man should have the prostate exam. High risk groups include men with history of prostate cancer in their family. **African-American men** should start having this yearly exam from age 40.

PROSTATE CHECK UP

A check up is merely an office visit where your doctor gets your complete medical history including present symptoms, medical conditions or surgical procedures in the past, medication in use, and drug allergies. A family history of prostate cancer in close relatives is also noted since this type of cancer in a father or brother increase the chances of your having the disease.

Three-fourths of all prostate cancers are located at the back part of the prostate, which lies next to the rectum. A digital rectal examination of this area will enable your physician to feel any abnormality in the size, shape and firmness of your prostate. This exam is quick, simple, and an economical first step in diagnosis.

Q. How is the digital rectal exam performed?

Most men know of this exam; it is the object of many jokes. The patient is asked to undress from the waist down and bend over while standing next to an examining table. The physician lubricates a gloved finger and passes it gently in the rectum from which the prostate gland can be felt. Abnormalities in the rectum can also be checked at the same time. (It doesn't hurt!)

This digital exam however, is only 35% to 50% reliable in the detection of prostate cancer. Cancers situated further inside the prostate are difficult to detect with this method alone. If your doctor finds any changes in the size, shape, or firmness of the prostate from his digital exam, a **PSA** test (blood test for the detection of cancer) accompanies it. If your PSA test is abnormal, an **ultrasound exam** of the prostate will be recommended for further evaluation.

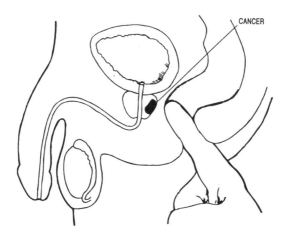

Digital Rectal Examination

Q. When is Ultrasound necessary?

Let's say the digital rectal examination and PSA **strongly suggest** the presence of disease. Then, your physician will probably recommend *ultrasound* (picture of the prostate generated by ultrasound echoes to detect the presence of cancer) and a biopsy of the prostate to confirm the diagnosis. Ultrasound is generally not recommended as a routine examination or a screening test because of the expense.

Q. What is involved in ultrasound and biopsy of the prostate?

A biopsy with the use of ultrasound is usually carried out in your physician's office and does not require anesthesia. You will be asked to eat a very light supper the night before the procedure and use a cleansing enema in the morning. Antibiotics an hour before the biopsy and for three days following will help prevent infections.

During the procedure itself, the patient lies on his side on the examining table. Then, an ultrasound transducer will be gently introduced into the rectum. Ultrasonic pictures will then show your doctor the prostate and surrounding area. If the ultrasound examination shows any abnormalities, a biopsy will be necessary.

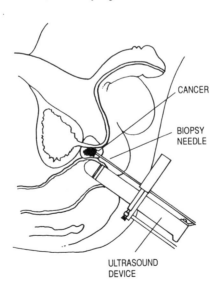

Trans-Rectal Ultrasound and Guided Biopsy of the Prostate

Q. What does a biopsy entail?

Often your doctor will take **six** biopsy samples of prostate tissue from different areas of the gland. Using a spring-loaded needle which goes through the ultrasound transducer, samples are quickly removed to minimize discomfort. Normally, this procedure takes 15 minutes.

Q. What does a biopsy reveal?

First, a biopsy of the prostate tissue reveals the presence or **absence** of cancer. Next, if cancer is found, a microscopic examination of the biopsy determines the **severity** or the **grade** of the cancer. Biopsy material can also be used to measure the DNA content which is yet another test to indicate the severity of the cancer.

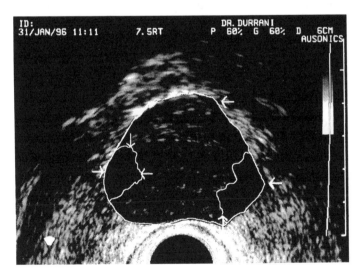

Ultrasound of the Prostate

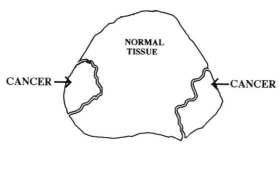

Prostate

Q. What exactly is PSA?

Prostate Specific Antigen (**PSA**) is a substance produced exclusively by the prostate and detectable in the blood. The normal, healthy prostate secretes PSA into the blood stream within a 0 to 4 ng/ml range. If a PSA test confirms **higher levels** than this in the blood, it could be due to an enlarged but benign prostate, a cancer of the prostate, or an inflammation of the prostate. Further evaluation will determine which one of these conditions is actually responsible for the elevation of PSA.

For instance, cancer of the prostate produces *ten times more* **PSA** than the healthy prostate; a PSA level that is high (over 10 ng/ml) may indicate a 60% to 90% probability of cancer. Usually the higher the PSA levels, the more extensive the cancer. However, cancer is not always associated with elevated PSA; 25% of cancers are found when PSA levels are within normal range.

PSA LEVELS ADJUSTED FOR AGE
Normal PSA ranges vary in different age groups

Age	40-49	50-59	60-69	70-79
PSA	0-2.5	0-3.5	0-4.5	0-6.5

PSA Density—A large but healthy prostate would produce a **higher level** of PSA than a small one. The same level in a small gland, however, may indicate trouble. Therefore, PSA levels must be considered in combination with the digital exam and ultrasound results to enable your doctor to calculate PSA values per cubic centimeter of prostate (called PSA density or **PSAD**).

PSA Velocity—Is the rate at which PSA level increases. Increasing PSA velocity may indicate progression in the growth of cancer. Increases in PSA velocity of 0.75 ng/ml per year for three years is strongly predictive of prostate cancer.

PSA-Free and Bound—When there is a moderate (between 4-10ng/ml) elevation of PSA, it is difficult to know if it is due to cancer or the benign enlargement of the prostate. If the PSA is further broken into its two fractions, namely, *free PSA* and *bound PSA*, diagnosis can be more precise.

Benign Prostatic Enlargement—causes elevation of the *free* PSA; whereas, **prostate cancer** causes elevation of the *bound* PSA.

I don't want to (further) confuse you with medical terminology you could care less about and, if you're not in the medical field, probably won't understand. Just feel confident that your urologist knows when to take additional tests to determine exactly the grade of cancer you might have so that the proper treatment can be prescribed. Each test brings both doctor and patient closer to the actual severity, if any, of this cancer.

PREVENTION
"An ounce of prevention is worth a pound of cure."

We have heard this parable since we were children. We heard it and we understand it, we've even quoted it. But, do we do anything about it? Usually we ignore it until *we* have it. In this instance we are talking about prostate cancer. Remember, more than *a third of a million* American men are diagnosed with prostate cancer each year. And, over 40,000 **die** because of it! Let's talk about prevention.

Vitamin D: In the laboratory, vitamin D has been shown to **suppress the growth** of prostate cancer cells, and it has also been suggested that vitamin D prevents the unimportant, inactive cancers from changing into **aggressive cancers**. Casual exposure to the sun allows the synthesis of vitamin D in the skin. As stated earlier, in Japan where the traditional diet is rich in **vitamin D** from fish, incidences of prostate cancer are LOW. In Scandinavian countries, where exposure to **SUNLIGHT** is low, mortality from prostate cancer is HIGH.

Vitamin A: Reports on the effectiveness of vitamin A in the reductions of prostate cancer risk are conflicting. Although either natural or synthetic vitamin A may reduce the risk of cancer to the lungs, larynx, cervix, and bladder, definitive studies of vitamin A and prostate cancer are needed and are not yet available.

Smoking: Some studies have suggested that cigarette smoking **increases** the risk of developing prostate cancer. The studies, however, are conflicting and the exact relation of smoking with prostate cancer is not clear. *Still, smoking is not good for health!*

Vasectomy: Some studies have it that risks of developing prostate cancer is higher in men who had undergone vasectomy. Relative risk of 1.5 to 2.2 has been reported; the risk increased with time after the vasectomy. There are also studies that found **no increase** in the risk of prostate cancer after vasectomy. A special panel at *the United States National Health Institute* concluded the available evidence was insufficient to support a clear conclusion at this time. The following

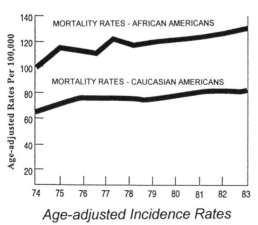

Age-adjusted Incidence Rates

three graphs show the age-adjusted incidence rates, and the age-adjusted mortality rate between African-Americans and Caucasian-Americans as well as the death rate in various countries.

If you are detected with having prostate cancer, there is no need to panic. Some prostate cancers are small and inactive, and may stay harmless throughout your life. But,

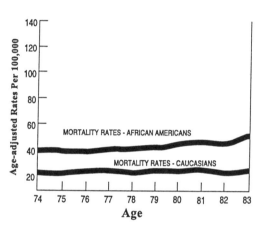

Prostate Cancer in Americans

once discovered during a routine screening, the majority of these cases need to be diagnosed with further tests. If it is detected early, your chances of **curative treatment** multiply greatly.

In Europe, routine screening is strongly opposed. In Canada, the Canadian Task Force on the Periodic Health Examination recommends no screening for prostate cancer in men without symptoms. Over diagnosis of potentially unimportant cancers and the cost of treatment are the two main objections to routine screening.

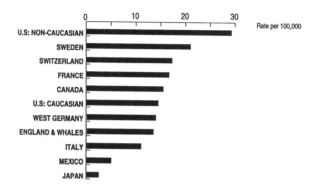

Prostate Cancer in Selected Countries

      70% to 90% of prostate cancers detected at a **routine screening** are still localized to the prostate, and potentially curable. Therefore, detection in men whose life expectancy is more than ten years can save their life. For instance, if a man is in his late seventies or early eighties, cancer in it's early stages will, undoubtedly, not be the cause of death. This cancer grows silently so that 45% of cases show no symptoms at the time of diagnosis.

      The risk of detecting unimportant cancers through prostate screening in normal men **without symptoms** is only 8%. This figure is in line with the risk of detecting unimportant cancers when patients come to the physician **with symptoms** and therefore does not represent an excessive or extraordinary risk.

Part 2

Extent of Prostate Cancer

In the past, many Americans have ignored the warnings, neglected to have a yearly physical exam, and felt that whatever it was that bothered them was slight and would go away. Not taking the opportunity to be tested for **early detection,** they now have advanced, ***metastasized*** (cancer that is malignant and spreading) cancer they are still unaware of. That yearly physical exam should be one of your top priorities! If you detect any of the following symptoms, consult your physician immediately.

SYMPTOMS OF ADVANCED CANCER

Anemia—Is a deficiency of blood which gives feelings of weakness and fatigue. Due to the destruction of bone marrow by invading cancer, the production of red blood cells decreases.

Treatment: Temporary relief of symptoms can be achieved through blood transfusions.

Swelling of the Legs—Is due to a blockage of the lymphatic vessels, which drain fluid from the veins in the legs. Then, fluid starts to accumulate and the legs swell. This condition is not really painful, but recovery is difficult.

Treatment: We use either **Hormone Therapy,**

where the use of hormones treats the cancer, or **Chemotherapy,** where the use of drugs **destroys** cancer cells. Each can reduce the size of the tumor and relieve compression on the veins and lymphatics.

Loss of Kidney Function—Due to cancer spread, the *ureters* become blocked and shut off the kidneys. Urine output ceases and the waste products accumulating in the body become toxic (*uremia*) causing drowsiness and coma.

      Treatment: A blockage of the *ureters* can be relieved surgically, but sometimes kidney dialysis is necessary first to flush the toxins from the body.

Spinal Cord Compression—It begins when the legs weaken, and later, complete paralysis develops. When the spinal cord is involved in the spread of the cancer, the nerves of the spinal cord become damaged. The nerves to the bladder may stop functioning and paralyze the bladder. This causes difficulty in urination and retention of urine occurs.

      Treatment: Radiation Therapy to destroy the cancer cells, and surgical **removal of the *testes*** can bring relief. A catheter can be used to empty the bladder in these cases.

Bone Pain and Bone Fractures—Due to involvement of the bones, fractures and pain may occur. *Metastastic* cancer starts to grow in the bones which cause bone **pains.** When cancer weakens the bones it can produce bone **fractures**.

Treatment: Radiation Therapy usually gives some relief from pain. Fractures may require surgery.

STAGES, GRADES and SPREAD of CANCER

Q. What exactly IS cancer?

Cancer is composed of **abnormal cells** which grow more rapidly than the normal cells and penetrate into the surrounding tissues. They spread into different parts of the body and eventually become lethal.

Q. What is the growth pattern of prostate cancer?

Prostate cancer may **stay dormant** for many years without any ill effect on health, or **may grow aggressively** with a fatal outcome. In general, the growth rate of prostate cancer is much slower than most other cancers. In the early stages, the cancer may take at least two years to double its size. Small cancers, below 0.5cc in volume, may be considered clinically harmless.

Q. What are the stages of prostate cancer?

The term *stage* of the cancer means the **extent** of the cancer, how large it is and how it is spreading. There are two systems of staging cancer of the prostate. The *Whitmore-Jewett* system is simple and the most commonly used that classifies prostate cancer into four main stages, namely A, B, C and D. Stage A being the least extensive and Stage D the most extensive cancer.

Let's describe the stages:

STAGE A CANCER . . . .
Is diagnosed unexpectedly when surgery is performed on an apparently benign enlarged prostate to relieve obstruction, and cannot be detected on Digital Rectal Examination. Stage A Cancers are further classified into **A$_1$** when the cancer is small *less than 5% of the tissue* and **A$_2$** when the cancer is *more than 5% of the tissue.*

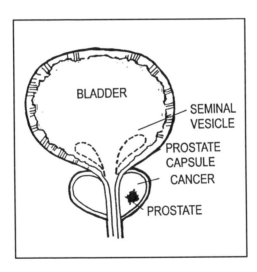

Stage A of Prostate Cancer

STAGE B CANCER . . . .
Is confined to the prostate. In substage **B$_1$,** the cancer is *smaller* than 1.5 cm and limited to a single lobe of the

prostate. In substage **B₂,** the cancer is either *larger* than 1.5 cm or involves *both* lobes of the prostate.

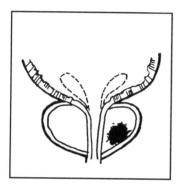

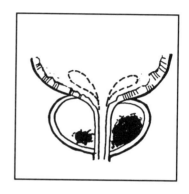

Stage B₁ of Prostate Cancer   *Stage B₂ of Prostate Cancer*

STAGE C CANCER . . . .

Extends *beyond* the capsule of the prostate.

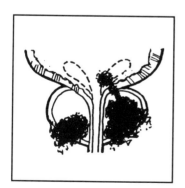

Stage C of Prostate Cancer

STAGE D CANCER . . . .
Means the cancer has spread beyond the prostate. There
are four parts of Stage D cancer:

D_0 is when the only indication of cancer spread
is the elevation of acid phosphatase on blood tests. D_1
means the cancer has spread to the lymph nodes in the
pelvis. D_2 *is* when the cancer has *metastasized* to the
bones. D_3 cancer *resists* cures by Hormone Treatment.

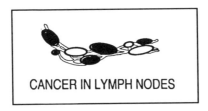

CANCER IN LYMPH NODES

Stage D_1 of Prostate Cancer

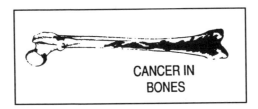

CANCER IN
BONES

Stage D_2 of Prostate Cancer

The above system to define cancer stages is
gradually being replaced by the more elaborate,
international classification called TNM—*Tumor, Node,
Metastasis* system. It describes the actual *size* of the

tumor, the **lymph node** involvement, and the **metastasis** (*spread*) if present.

T_0, no evidence of a tumor. T_1 is a tumor found unexpectedly on removal of prostate tissue for presumably benign enlargement of the prostate. It also cannot be detected on Digital Rectal Examination or on Imaging (X-ray).

T_2 is a tumor confined within the prostate. The three substages are:

> T_{2a} involves a tumor that is half or less of one lobe of the prostate.
>
> T_{2b} means that the tumor is in *more than half* of a single lobe but not in both lobes.
>
> T_{2c} involves a tumor in **both lobes.**

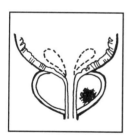   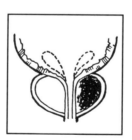   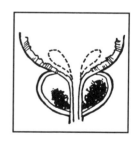

Stage T_{2a} Stage T_{2b} Stage T_{2c}

T_3 is a tumor that extends *through* the capsule of the prostate. The substages are:

> T_{3a} extends through the capsule on **one** side
>
> T_{3b} extends through on **both** sides.
>
> T_{3c} involves seminal vesicles.

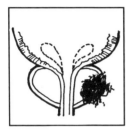 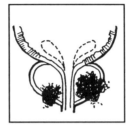 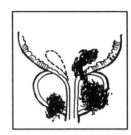

Stage T$_{3a}$ *Stage T$_{3b}$*   *Stage T$_{3c}$*

T$_4$ is a tumor that invades surrounding structures other than the seminal vesicles. **T$_4$** substages are:

> **T$_{4a}$** is when the tumor invades the bladder neck and/or external sphincter and/or rectum.
>
> **T$_{4b}$** is when it invades the levator muscles and/or fixed to the pelvic wall.

T$_x$, *primary tumor cannot be assessed.*

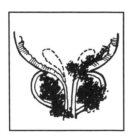 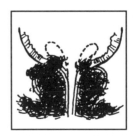

Stage T$_{4a}$ of Prostate Cancer   *Stage T$_{4b}$ of Prostate Cancer*

LYMPH NODE INVOLVEMENT . . . .

N_o, regional lymph nodes not involved. N_1, Metastasis (spread) in a single regional lymph node (2 or less). N_2, Spread in a single regional lymph node, but between 2.5 cm in diameter or multiple regional lymph nodes, none more than 5 cm. N_3, Spread (metastasis) in regional lymph nodes more than 5 cm in size. N_x, regional lymph nodes cannot be assessed.

METASTASIS . . . .

By now and throughout the book you'll see this word which simply means **spread.** M_o, no distant spread. M_1 means distant spread is present.

M_{1a} signifies lymph node involvement *outside* regional zones.

M_{1b} means spread to the bones.

M_{1c} the cancer has spread to *other sites.*

M_x distant spread cannot be assessed.

I'd like to tell you something about these stages and explanations. If you are a patient, your urologist will certainly explain them to you and this book is of little benefit other than to aid you in recalling the terminology. It does, however, serve as a reminder of the severity of this disease and will hopefully prompt you to schedule an exam to detect prostate cancer before it gets into any of the latter stages.

It is also helpful, I feel, for those who have a loved one who has prostate cancer, for them to understand the treatments, complications and severity of the disease in these various stages. Now, let's find out more.

Q. How does prostate cancer spread?

The prostate is enclosed within its capsule. Cancer is initially confined within the capsule which provides some resistance to its spread. As the tumor grows, however, it penetrates through the capsule. The cancer can spread locally and to distant organs.

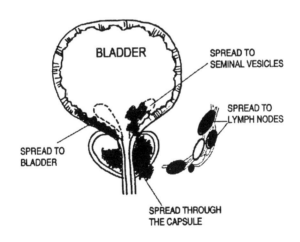

Local Spread

Q. What do you mean by Local Spread?

After penetrating through the capsule, the cancer may invade *seminal vesicles, bladder, neck* and the surrounding other tissues. Once the disease has spread to this extent, the prognosis is poor. Invasion of the *ureters* obstructs urine flow from the kidneys resulting in life-threatening *uremia* (accumulation of toxins waste-products of the body).

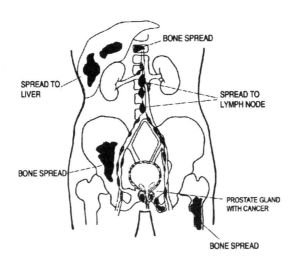

Distant Spread Of Cancer

Q. What is Lymphatic Spread?

Spread to the *lymph nodes* usually occurs in larger and in very aggressive cancers. At first, the local *pelvic lymph nodes* are involved; later, the distant *lymph nodes* in the abdomen, chest and the neck are affected.

Q. How does it spread through the blood stream?

If prostate cancer spreads through the blood stream, it will commonly involve the bones of the pelvis, spine, ribs and femur. Other organs such as the lungs, liver, and the adrenal glands become involved in the late stages of prostate cancer.

Q. What are the different grades of cancer?

The severity of a malignancy is determined by examining the cancer cells under a microscope. A grade or score is then determined based on the abnormality of the architecture of the cells, abnormality of the nucleus, and the extent of the invasion into the surrounding tissues. Although a completely reliable system of grading this cancer has not been found, the system used most often is the *Gleason Grading System, where* scores of 2-4 refers to low grade cancers which are the least malignant; conversely, Gleason scores of 7-10 indicates high-grade cancers with very poor prognosis.

Q. What is Prostatic Intraepithelial Neoplasia (PIN)?

A malignancy which is limited to the cells of the lining of the microscopic gland *acini,* and does not yet invade the deeper tissues. Because PIN does not invade tissues, it does not spread or cause any ill effects. This type of limited cancer is classified as a **low-grade PIN**, usually not significant, or a **high-grade PIN**, the more worrisome condition.

A high grade PIN may be associated with a definite, **invasive cancer** lying next to it in the prostate, or it may change into one. A high grade PIN needs to be watched closely and monitored with periodic biopsies.

Q. What is DNA Ploidy?

Ploidy refers to the amount of DNA in the nucleus of a cell. Cancer cells have higher content of DNA in their nucleus as compared to the normal cells. DNA content or *DNA Ploidy* is higher in cancers with a high grade of malignancy. Normal DNA content is called *diploid*: the higher content can be *tetraploid* or *aneuploid*. The prognosis is poor in cancers with high DNA content.

TESTS FOR STAGES OF CANCER

To determine the extent of cancer, before surgery, you may expect your doctor to use some of the following diagnostic studies.

Prostate Specific Antigen (PSA): We mentioned this earlier on in the text when we talked of preliminary testing. Remember, it helps detect cancer and is one of the initial tests to determine whether surgery is necessary? PSA is a substance produced exclusively from the prostate. High value of PSA in the blood is due to the large size of the prostate, inflammation, and cancer of the prostate.

Prostate Acid Phosphatase (PAP): A blood test similar to PSA but less sensitive. High values of this PAP may indicate the presence of advanced cancer.

Transrectal Ultrasound: Simply a *camera-like* instrument that transmits and receives echoes that detect the presence of cancer.

Prostate Biopsy: A specimen removed from the tissue for microscopic examination.

Bone Scan: A picture of the skeleton taken after intravenous administration of nuclear material. Cancer deposits in the bone show abnormally a high intake of the nuclear material.

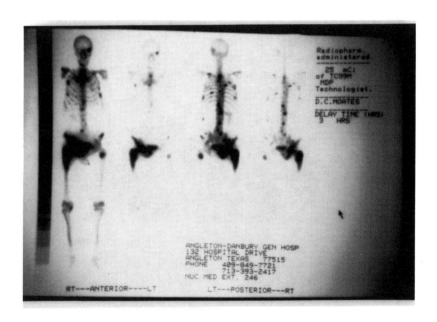

The Dark Areas Depict Cancer

CAT Scan of Pelvis: I know most of you have heard of this, well this is what it is. **CAT Scan** stands for *Computer Assisted Tomography SCAN* that gives X-ray images in more than a one dimensional view

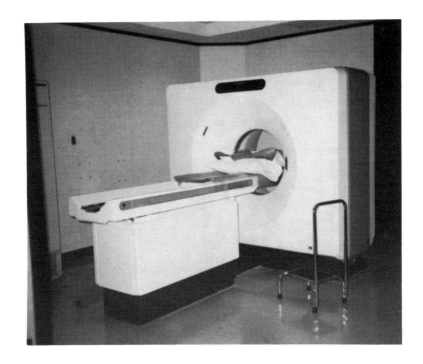

Cat Scan

Magnetic Resonance Imaging (MRI): You're probably aware of this terminology too. The MRI takes images of the body by modern resonance technique instead of X-rays.

The **final** confirmation that the cancer has not spread outside the prostate is only possible when the *pelvic lymph nodes* have been examined. A biopsy of the pelvic nodes is obtained by open surgery or through laparoscopic technique.

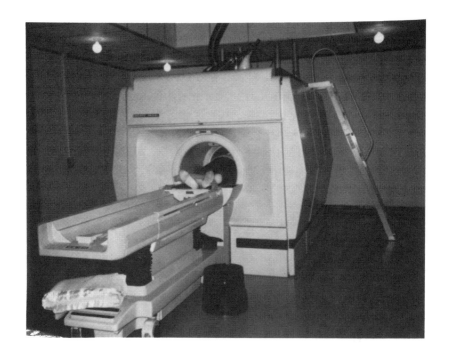

MRI

Q. Is it necessary to use ALL of these methods to detect cancer?

Yes! Each test is helpful and essential in determining stages and severity of cancer.

Q. How do I prepare myself for surgery if I need it?

A week before scheduled surgery you will need to **discontinue** using aspirin and other **anti-inflammatory** drugs which interfere with blood clotting. In the event a transfusion becomes necessary during surgery, you might want to reserve one or two pints of your own blood. Many people prefer using their own blood for fear of HIV or Hepatitis. If more blood is needed, it can be obtained from a blood bank.

You'll also need **Lab Tests**, where blood will be drawn for routine preoperative tests and a chest X-ray and EKG will be ordered to make sure your lungs and heart are normal.

Then, for **Preoperative Preparation**, you will be asked for a complete medical history and given a physical. Antibiotics such as *Neomycin* and *Erythromycin* will also be prescribed the night before surgery to minimize bacterial contamination if the bowel is injured during the operation. A **cleansing enema** is given on the morning of surgery, which reduces the possibility of infection in the event of injury to the rectum.

Before the actual surgery you will confer with an *anesthesiologist* to decide whether you will be given a **General** anesthetic, which puts you completely asleep, or a **Regional** anesthetic, usually an epidural, anesthetizes (numbs) only the lower half of the body.

The catheter used for injecting epidural anesthetic is usually left in place for a few days after surgery for medications to control post operative pain. When pain is controlled, a patient can get out of bed early and some of the serious postoperative complications such as clotting of blood in the legs and pneumonia can be prevented.

Of course, you will have a conference with your

physician, to go over the surgical procedure and post-operative care. He will answer any questions you may have and explain what surgical approach he is going to use to remove the prostate.

Part 3

Surgical Options

For over 100 years, skilled physicians have recommended surgery in the treatment of prostate cancer. Surgical techniques have been refined to minimize blood loss and preserve the nerves responsible for sexual potency. Postoperative recovery has improved over the years as well, while complications have become fewer.

Q. When is surgery recommended?

When cancer is clinically confined to the prostate, the main concern for surgery is to completely **remove** the cancer for cure.

PELVIC LYMPH NODE DISSECTION

The tests that were performed that have led us to detect cancer do not give **absolute assurance** that the cancer has not spread to the lymph nodes. If this is the case, we begin with what is called **Pelvic Lymph Node Dissection.** Let me tell you about lymph nodes.

They are small structures varying from a few millimeters to a centimeter (not even a ½") into which lymphatic vessels drain lymphatic fluid. These lymph nodes trap bacteria and cancer cells and try to destroy them.

Therefore, before removing the prostate, your

urologist will take out these lymph nodes and rush them to the lab. In the lab, the nodes are frozen and thinly sliced into sections that can be examined under a microscope. A biopsy report is usually available in 30 minutes. If it shows cancer, surgery of the prostate is not the treatment. If the diagnosis is no cancer in the lymph nodes, the cancer is considered confined to the prostate which is then removed.

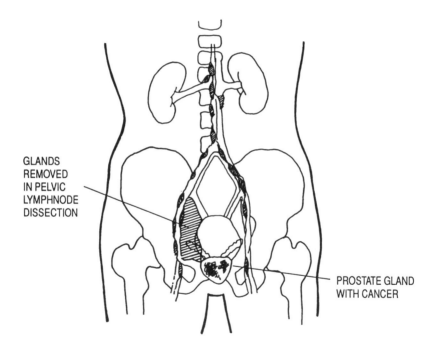

GLANDS
REMOVED
IN PELVIC
LYMPHNODE
DISSECTION

PROSTATE GLAND
WITH CANCER

Pelvic Lymph Node Dissection

LAPROSCOPIC PLN DISSECTION

There is another technique used to remove the *pelvic lymph nodes* for a biopsy by using a Laparoscope. **Laparoscopic Pelvic Lymph Node Dissection** is carried out with the patient under a general anesthesia, where the abdomen is inflated with carbon dioxide gas to allow room for the instruments to maneuver without injuring the bowel or other organs. Next, a small telescope, fitted out with a miniature high-resolution TV camera is inserted through a small incision in the abdominal wall. Using miniature instruments, the surgeon is able to dissect the tissues while viewing the internal area on a TV screen. **Laparoscopic Pelvic Lymph Node Dissection (LPLND)**, as it is called, has some advantages over removing the lymph nodes through an abdominal incision; the hospital stay is shorter (usually overnight) and the convalescence is faster.

The actual time of the laparoscopic procedure, however, is about twice as long (approximately three hours). Complications during this operation include risk of injury to abdominal organs such as perforation of the bowel, injury to the bladder or major blood vessels. (Laparoscopy is not suitable for obese patients or those who may have adhesions due to previous abdominal surgery).

There are two methods currently in use to operate on the prostate. The most common is:

RADICAL RETROPUBIC PROSTATECTOMY

The **Radical Retropubic Prostatectomy** involves making an incision in the lower abdomen from the navel to the pubic bone to reach the prostate and surgically, take it out. If your surgeon decides to use abdominal incision for the prostate surgery, pelvic lymph node dissection can be carried out through the same incision under the same anesthesia.

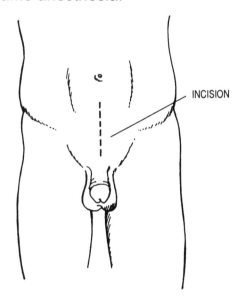

INCISION

Incision for Radical Retropubic Prostatectomy

When the results from the lab indicate that the prostate should be removed, the surgeon will begin to free the prostate from the surrounding tissues. The veins at the apex of the prostate are ligated to prevent bleeding, and the rectum at the back is carefully freed from the prostate gland.

The neurovascular bundles along the sides of the prostate are then carefully separated out in order to preserve the nerves responsible for erection. It is not always possible to save these nerves, particularly if the cancer is big or too close to the nerve bundles. The urethra is transected at the apex of the prostate. At the base of the prostate, the *bladder neck* is divided from the prostate, and finally, the *seminal vesicles* are removed along with the prostate itself.

The wide *bladder neck* is narrowed to match the size of the *urethra*. A catheter is inserted in the *urethra* and passed through the *bladder neck* into the bladder. With sutures, the *bladder neck* is joined with the *urethra* to reestablish the continuity of the urinary tract. The catheter is worn for 2 to 3 weeks until the junction is healed. Wearing a catheter is not usually painful, but it is cumbersome to carry the drainage bag around. For comfort and maneuverability, a small bag can be strapped to the leg and worn with loose clothing.

Presently, the abdominal incision technique is the most widely used procedure for **Radical Prostatectomy**. It has the advantage of combining lymph node removal and prostate removal through the same incision. A most significant advantage with this technique is that it allows your surgeon to better preserve the nerves which control **potency.**

RADICAL PERINEAL PROSTATECTOMY

A small semicircular incision is made between the scrotum and the rectum. This surgical approach which uses incision through the *perineum* is the older of the two methods. It had gone out of favor for a long time, but recently, it has been gaining interest among surgeons because it gives direct exposure of the operative field and makes certain steps of surgery easier to perform. Blood loss is less during the *perineal* approach, but it has the disadvantage of requiring a separate procedure to remove the lymph nodes (usually a laparoscopic procedure).

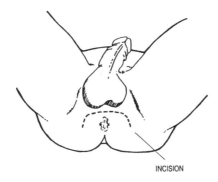

INCISION

Incision for Radical Perineal Prostatectomy

No matter which surgical technique is used, both entail a 4 to 7-day hospital stay. Stitches are removed after a week and the urethral catheter is removed two to three weeks after surgery.

SALVAGE SURGERY

Salvage Surgery is undertaken to remove local disease in the patients who have failed radiation therapy. The surgical procedure may be in the form of conventional **Radical Prostatectomy** (total removal of the prostate along with seminal vesicles) or it may involve removal of the bladder and rectum along with the prostate if the disease is extensive.

Technically, surgery of tissues which have been exposed to radiation is quite difficult and carries a high incidence of complications. Chances of complete removal of cancer are limited. The procedure may be used in young patients with low grade disease but it is not recommended as a routine procedure after failure of Radiation Therapy.

Q. What complications can result from surgery?

Blood loss during surgery is usually about 1-2 pints. Blood transfusions are not always necessary; however, your doctor will always want blood available in the event blood loss exceeds expectations. Before surgery you will be given the opportunity to donate one to two pints of your own blood (for those of you who are concerned about unknown or possible contaminated sources).

Blood clots in the veins have a tendency to develop in the legs or the pelvic veins. Besides causing swelling of the legs, the clots may dislodge and move to the heart or the brain causing life-threatening situations.

Your doctor will want you to begin standing and walking as soon as possible after surgery and ask you to wear elastic stockings to help prevent these complications due to clotting.

IMPOTENCE DISCUSSED IN PART 6

Incontinenceis the loss of urinary control after surgery can be due to irritability of the bladder. This kind of incontinence soon recovers as the inflammation of the bladder resolves. A more serious form of incontinence is due to weakness of the sphincter muscle caused by surgery. This type of incontinence occurs in about 5% of patients. When it is minor (only a few leaking drops now and then) it can be managed with protective pads.

Severe incontinence may need surgical procedure such as injection of collagen in the urethra or implantation of an artificial sphincter.

Injections of collagen through a *cystoscope* to narrow the bladder neck has also been helpful in recovering bladder control. Severe urinary incontinence may need surgical procedure to implant an artificial sphincter.

A **rectal injury** can be a serious complication of Radical Prostatectomy and will require a repair of the laceration and a course of antibiotics to control infection.

Lymphocele (a collection of fluid leaking from the lymphatic vessels) can also appear after surgery. Usually this condition resolves itself on its own; larger lymphocele may require drainage.

Part 4

Methods Other Than Surgery

RADIATION THERAPY

This type of therapy has been used in the treatment of prostate cancer since the beginning of this century. Radiation injures or kills the targeted cancerous cells or disrupts their ability to reproduce causing them to eventually disappear. Technical advances and clinical experience have greatly improved this treatment.

Q. When is Radiation Therapy recommended?

When the cancer is still confined to the prostate! Radiation Therapy is more suitable for patients who are **over the age of early seventies** or **who cannot tolerate surgery due to poor general health**. It is also a treatment choice for the patients who are not prepared to accept the risks of possible complications of surgery.

Radiation Therapy is also used in the treatment of locally extensive cancer which cannot be removed completely with surgery. In such cases radiation therapy can be used either exclusively or in conjunction with *Hormone Therapy*, or after surgery. It is also sometimes used in advanced disease to relieve bone pains from metastastic spread of prostate cancer.

Q. Is Pelvic Lymph Node Dissection necessary before

Radiation Therapy?

It is important to know that cancer has not spread to the lymph nodes before deciding to use radiation therapy. In low grade cancers and where PSA elevation is minor, the chances of lymph node involvement are very low. Such patients can be spared the procedure of lymph node dissection with presumption that cancer is most likely confined to the prostate.

However, patients with **high grade cancer** or those who have PSA values of more than 20ng/ml are very likely to have *metastastic* disease in the pelvic lymph nodes. In such patients, it is recommended that Pelvic Lymph Node Dissection be carried out. If the lymph nodes show cancer, the patient would not be benefited by radiation therapy and would be better treated with hormone therapy.

Pelvic Lymph Node Dissection before Radiation Therapy can be carried out through *laparoscopic* technique, or through a small incision in the lower abdomen, so-called **minilap** (small *laparotomy)* incision.

Q. How is Radiation Therapy delivered?

There are two methods; the first, *Local Irradiation* (*brachytherapy),* is when radioactive material is implanted directly into the tissue of the prostate. Originally, implantation entailed a fairly major surgical procedure through an incision in the lower abdomen. Today, by using ultrasound technology, it is possible to guide a needle through the perineal area and implant the radioactive material without an incision.

The main benefit of *Brachytherapy* is that a comparatively large dose of radiation can be delivered locally with minimal radiation effects on the surrounding normal tissue; the main drawback is that the radiation is not evenly distributed in the cancer, thus, some of the cancer may survive.

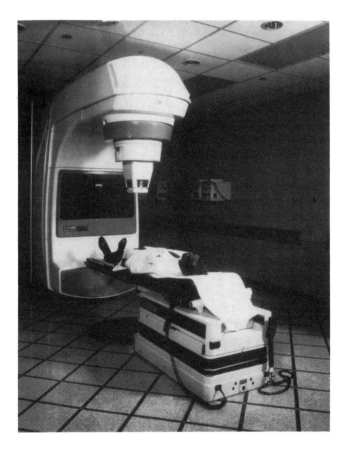

External Beam Radiation

The second method is ***External Beam Irradiation,*** a more widely used method of delivering radiation. The most commonly used source of energy for teletherapy is high-energy X-rays enhanced by a 6 to 25-megavolt linear accelerators.

In this method, radiation is directed at the prostate from the **front, back, right and left sides** of the pelvis. CAT scans and treatment simulators are used to locate the target and direct the beam precisely. The boundaries of the field are carefully shielded so that the surrounding organs (particularly the rectum, anal canal, and small bowel) are protected from radiation.

A total dose is calculated (usually 6,000 to 7,000 cGy) and the treatment is spread over a period of 6-8 weeks. Although the first treatment may require some time in mapping out the site and programming the dosages, treatments thereafter will only take a few minutes to painlessly deliver the prescribed radiation dose.

Q. What complications are possible with Radiation Therapy?

With advanced technology and extensive clinical experience the complications of Radiation Therapy have greatly decreased. Generally, the rate of developing complications is related to the **radiotherapy** technique and to the total radiation dose; a high total dose of radiation (more than 7,000 cGy) significantly increases the incidence of complications. Here are some of the most general problems after Radiation Therapy.

Impotence

Sexual impotence is not an infrequent complication of *External Beam Radiation Therapy*. In a report of 133 patients treated with external beam irradiation, 29% of the patients who had been potent before the treatment complained of impotence following treatment.

Urinary Complications

Urinary complications are relatively infrequent, occurring in about 7-8% of cases treated with radiation; most of these are of moderate severity and resolve without treatment. A common urinary complication is bladder inflammation (*cystitis*) which gives symptoms of discomfort or pain and frequency in urination.

Only 0.5% of the patients experience severe complications including *hematuria* (blood in the urine), strictures of urethra, or contracture of the bladder. These problems can be controlled with transfusion or surgery. Urinary complications may take several months to develop and can occur from 3-18 months after therapy.

Rectal Complications

Rectal complications occur even less frequently than urinary complications as a result of Radiation Therapy. A common rectal complication is rectal inflammation (*proctitis)* which causes symptoms of diarrhea, rectal discomfort, and frequent bowel movements. In a large study of 1,020 patients treated with External Beam Radiation, rectal complications occurred in only 3.3% of the cases.

Most symptoms experienced by patients were only moderately severe; however, there were two deaths: one from rectal bleeding and one from an intestinal obstruction. Rectal complications may take from several months to years to develop after therapy.

Other Complications

Leg and scrotal swelling are the least common of the complications, occurring in less than 1% of all cases. Elastic stockings and leg elevation after surgery can remedy minor swelling problems.

Q. How often will I need to come in for follow-up exams after radiation therapy?

This varies with physicians, but generally a patient is seen every two to three months during the first year after therapy, and at three to six months intervals thereafter. These visits include routine blood work, a PSA, a urinalysis, and a digital rectal examination. The PSA is the most valuable tool for evaluating the result of the treatment. In the first three to six months after radiation therapy, the PSA should gradually fall, coming to normal values within the first year in favorable cases.

Because the prostate is not removed in Radiation Therapy, unlike surgical treatment, the prostate is still capable of producing PSA. Elevation of PSA can predict recurrence 1-3½ years sooner than any other method of diagnosis. If the PSA is elevated and *metastasis* is suspected, a bone scan is carried out for confirmation.

Q. What happens if I experience a relapse after Radiation Therapy?

A failure of the radiation treatment may appear as a local recurrence or metastastic spreading. Failure of treatment is indicated by rising PSA or evidence of cancer on re-biopsy of the prostate 18 months or more after radiation therapy. In patients for which Radiation Therapy has failed, Hormone Therapy, Cryosurgery, or Salvage Surgery may be considered.

Q. What are the survival rates with Radiation Therapy?

Biologically, more aggressive tumors have a poor prognosis compared to less aggressive tumors. The results of Radiation Therapy depend largely on the extent or clinical stage of the tumor. In a large series of 1,119 patients treated with external beam radiation, patients in an early stage of cancer (Stage **A**) had a 15-year survival rate which is similar to that normally expected for men in that age group. However, when the patients were not treated until more advanced stages, the 15-year survival rate fell to 20-30%.

Q. How does Radiation Therapy compare with surgical treatment?

Radiation Therapy and surgery both aim at curing *localized* prostate cancer. In comparing the two methods, the benefits of each need to be weighed against the potential complications. Generally, Radiation Therapy is preferable for patients who are **seventy** or older, are a poor surgical risk due to general health, or wish to avoid the potential surgical complications.

A review of a series of case histories showed that the 10-year survival rate was better (93%) in patients who underwent *Radical Prostatectomy* than in those who were treated with Radiation Therapy (73%). It is important to note that these studies may have selected patients with less severe cases of cancer for surgery and, physicians' recommendation can have personal bias.

In another study, physicians were asked which form of treatment they would choose for themselves if they had cancer of the prostate; most urologists chose **surgery,** and most radiation oncologist chose **Radiation Therapy**. Without hard and fast guidelines or recommendations stemming from adequate clinical trials, one must depend largely on personal feelings and individual circumstances when deciding.

Q. What is Strontium-89?

It is a *radioisotope,* and like calcium it is preferentially taken up by the bones. It concentrates in the bones, especially in the *metastastic* cancer deposits, where it delivers its radiation.

It is also used for the relief of pain from the metastastic deposits of cancer in the bones. It has been reported to be effective in relieving bone pains in up to 80% of the patients. It is given in the form of an intravenous injection, as an outpatient treatment. The radiation effect of *Strontium-89* lasts a long time so that the dose does not have to be repeated for 2 to 3 months. The **side effect** of *Strontium-89* is mainly from its toxic effect on the bone marrow.

The bone marrow reduces production of blood cells and platelets which are necessary for the normal blood clotting mechanism in the body. This may result in a tendency to bleed. A periodic blood count is carried out to assess the toxic effects on the marrow.

WATCHFUL WAITING

Q. When is *Watchful Waiting* recommended?

Watchful Waiting has no place in treatment of most cancers, however, **prostate cancer** is an exception. In some cases where the cancer is localized to the prostate, where the patient is in poor health, or far advanced in years, monitoring and waiting before further, more aggressive steps are taken can be justified until the disease starts to show progression.

Although the object of treating *any* cancer is to completely eradicate the disease, in the treatment of prostate cancer, removing the cancer is not obligatory for a 10 to 15-year survival. The growth rate of prostate cancer is so slow that it takes several years for the initial cancer to grow large enough to penetrate the capsule and spread outside the prostate.

During this time, before *metastasis* occurs, the cancer may have no deleterious effect on health. In fact, most of these cancers are never even diagnosed and **remain harmless** and **undetected** throughout life. In view of such slow growth it is often debatable whether a **localized cancer** of the prostate should be treated aggressively with surgery or watched closely to see if it progresses. In fact, potential complications of surgery or Radiation Therapy on the quality of life may outweigh the benefit of an extended life span.

Opponents of *Watchful Waiting* maintain that a cure is only possible with aggressive treatment, and that waiting denies the patient of this opportunity. After successful surgical removal of a cancer in a man of 65 or younger, the 15-year survival rate is the same as that expected in normal men of that age. Risks of complications remain, but recent advances in surgical techniques have reduced the rate significantly.

Q. Are there guidelines in deciding to Watch and Wait?

The following guidelines should be considered when you make the decision either to wait, or to pursue more aggressive treatment.

Extent of the Cancer
Small cancers progress very slowly allowing a long period of time before any deleterious effect occurs on health.

Aggressiveness of the Cancer
As judged by its microscopic appearance, it is closely related to the rate of progression and prognosis. Because **low grade cancers progress slowly**, survival can be 10 times longer in a low grade cancer than the highly aggressive type. The option of Watchful Waiting may be justified in low grade cancers which are likely to be

harmless for long time.

Age
Watchful waiting is more suitable for older men (mid-seventies), who have a life expectancy of 10 years or less since prostate cancer would often progress very slowly. In younger men however, aggressive treatment promises a good possibility of completely eradicating the disease and might be more desirable than having to deal with the eventual progression of the disease under Watchful Waiting.

General Health
For patients who have poor general health (diseases of the heart, lungs) or other serious physical conditions may make some patients unsuitable for **aggressive** treatment.

The patient and the physician together should make the final decision. At present, unfortunately, there is not enough clinical data[1] available to strongly recommend either treatment. The benefits of each treatment have

---

Further studies are needed to evaluate the pros and cons of the different treatment methods. One such study, sponsored by the Veterans Administration and the National Cancer Institute, is now in progress. Prostate Cancer Intervention Versus Observation Trial (PIVOT), as the project is called, is a controlled study in which 2,000 patients will be followed-up for 12 years to monitor treatments. Results of this study are expected to make valuable recommendations in the choice of treatment of early stage prostate cancer.

to be weighed against the possible risks on an individual basis.

Q. What is entailed in Watchful Waiting?

During Watchful Waiting regimen, the patient is assessed on regular intervals. Clinical signs of progression of the disease are checked by monitoring PSA levels. Repeat biopsy, bone scan, and CAT scan or MRI may be needed. When progression is noticed, there may still be a small chance of aggressive treatment such as surgery or radiation treatment; otherwise, Hormone Therapy is started.

HORMONE THERAPY

Q. Talk about Hormone Therapy.

The concept of treating prostate cancer with Hormone Therapy began in 1941 when Huggins and Hodges demonstrated dramatic improvement in prostate cancer patients when their *testes* were **surgically removed** to stop the production of the male hormone *testosterone*. In 1966, Charles Huggins received the Noble Prize for his work on Hormone Therapy.

Q. When is Hormone Therapy recommended?

In advanced cancer of the prostate when a cure is not possible with surgery or Radiation Therapy. It is also employed after surgery, or when Radiation Therapy, or Watchful Waiting fails and progression of the disease is suspected.

Q. How does Hormone Therapy work?

Testosterone is essential for the normal growth and development of the prostate. Boys who are *eunuchs* (when the *testes* are absent at birth) in childhood show arrested growth of the prostate gland. Because cancer of the prostate also requires *testosterone*, these boys will run very little risk of developing this disease in later life. When *testosterone* is withdrawn from the body by surgically removing the *testes* or blocking the action of the hormone by drugs, the prostate cancer cells begin to die.

Q. What is Surgical Orchiectomy?

The most well-known name for it is **castration!** A modern surgical removal of the *testes*, or **Orchiectomy**, is the oldest method for removing *testosterone* in the body. Despite the availability of potent drugs which can produce this same effect, **Surgical Orchiectomy** continues to be a viable treatment due to its lower cost and its surgical simplicity (usually done as an outpatient procedure). Orchiectomy causes a marked reduction in the size of prostate cancer and has been shown to relieve urinary obstructions in almost 70% of the patients who experience urinary retention as a result of their cancer.

This procedure has also been proven to relieve bone pains due to *metastatic* cancer. Orchiectomy will cause a loss of *libido* and impotence, making it psychologically very difficult for patients (especially younger patients) to accept.

Q. What is Medical Castration?

Action of *testosterone* can also be blocked by medication achieving results similar to Surgical Castration. The drugs used for this Hormone Therapy are *estrogen*, *LHRH analogs, antiandrogens*, and certain other drugs.

Q. What is Estrogen?

A female hormone, usually administered orally in the form of *diethylstilbestrol* (DES). It has been used for many years in the treatment of **advanced cancer of the prostate.** Estrogen Therapy may cause significant side-effects however, including serious cardiovascular complications, enlargement of breasts (*gynecomastia),* loss of libido (sex drive), and impotence. Because of the potential side-effects, estrogen is now seldom used for the treatment of cancer of the prostate.

Q. What does LHRH stand for?

Luteinizing Hormone Releasing Hormones (LHRH) are normally produced in the *hypothalamus gland* in the brain. The function of LHRH is to stimulate the *pituitary gland* to produce *gonadotropic hormones* called LH, which in turn, stimulates the *testes* to produce *testosterone.* The aim of hormone treatment is to stop the production of *testosterone* which causes prostate cancer to grow.

Normally, LHRH release comes in pulses to stimulate the pituitary. If LHRH is released constantly and in excessive quantity (as in Hormone Therapy) it **suppresses the pituitary and stops LH production** which in turn causes the testes to stop producing testosterone. The two most widely used synthetic LHRHs in the U.S. are *Lupron®* and *Zoladex®*; both are in a slow-release form which allow one injection to last for a month. The newer injections now available have the drugs that last for three months. The results of treatment with LHRH are as good as with a surgical orchiectomy. Side-effects include the loss of libido, impotence and hot flashes.

ANTIANDROGENS

Q. What are Antiandrogens?

Antiandrogens are drugs which **inhibit** *testosterone* activity; the most commonly used in the US has been a nonsteroidal type called *Flutamide*.

Flutamide is commonly used in *metastastic* cancer of the prostate, in combination with surgical orchiectomy or LHRH therapy. It is administered orally and is generally well tolerated, although some gastrointestinal symptoms may occur in some cases. Severe side-effects, in the form of fatal and non-fatal liver toxicity have also been reported. A periodic check of the liver functions is helpful in detecting the toxicity.

Q. How about Bicalutamide?

Bicalutamide also has recently been approved by the Federal Drug Administration for use in advanced cancer of the prostate. It, too, is taken orally and has a convenient once-a-day dosage schedule. It has been used as a single agent or in combination with LHRH *agonist* drugs. It is generally well tolerated. The most frequent side effects are, enlargement of the breasts (*gynecomastia*), hot flashes, decreased libido and impotence.

Q. How about Nilutamide?

Another *nosteriodal antiandrogen* drug, available in tablet form to be taken by mouth. When used it LHRH therapy it will give a total androgen blockade.

Q. Tell me about Finasteride.

Finasteride (Proscar® , Merck and Co., Inc.) *is also an antiandrogen* . It is an oral medication that reduces the size of benign enlarged prostate and it also lowers PSA usually by 50%. Laboratory studies have shown that *Finasteride* **inhibits the growth** of cancer cells. Clinical studies are being carried out to find out if it can prevent or suppress prostate cancer.

Q. And Ketoconazole?

Ketoconazole was originally used as an antifungal drug. It was found to cause suppression of production of t*estosterone* both in the *testes* and the adrenal glands. It also has some **anti-cancer** properties, and is sometimes used in the treatment of *metastastic* cancer of the prostate when the usual hormone therapy fails. Its main side-effect is toxicity on the liver. When using this drug, liver functions need to be monitored with periodic blood tests.

Q. Please talk about timing of Hormone Therapy.

Although hormone treatment is used in *metastastic*

cancer of the prostate which is already an advanced stage of the disease, the term **early Hormone Therapy** refers to the treatment started soon after the diagnosis is made. The **delayed Hormone Therapy** is the treatment which is started when the disease becomes symptomatic or further progression is evident.

Advantages are documented in the literature in favor of the early hormone treatment in terms of **prolonging** symptom-free interval, **delaying** disease progression, **improving** quality of life and **increasing** survival rate.

However, there are certain **disadvantages** of Hormone Therapy which have to be weighed against the benefits of the early treatment. *Orchiectomy* involves surgical procedure, psychological trauma, loss of libido and impotence. LHRH analogues incur high cost of medication, hot flashes and impotence. Antiandrogens like *Flutamide* may give gastrointestinal symptoms and gynecomastia *(enlargement of breasts)*. This can occur in men receiving estrogens for the treatment of advanced cancer of the prostate. With delayed treatment, the potential disadvantages of Hormone Therapy are avoided until the treatment starts.

It may be preferable to hold off the early Hormone Therapy in a low grade cancer in an older patient who may never show any complication from the tumor during his life span. On the other hand in the younger patient, with a high grade tumor, **early Hormone Therapy** could **increase survival.** If the treatment is postponed for too long, it may become ineffective because **cancer becomes**

hormone-resistant in the late stages!

Q. What is Preoperative Hormone Therapy?

This has been used with the idea of reducing the extent (*down sizing*) of cancer so that it could be surgically removed completely without leaving any cancer tissue behind. **LHRH analogs, estrogens** or **Bilateral Orchiectomy** has been used for 3-6 months before surgery. Some beneficial effects have been seen but the results have not been consistently encouraging.

Q. Is Hormone Therapy effective in all patients?

Not all patients who have *metastastic* cancer of the prostate, but 60-80% initially show good response. Hormone Therapy causes an active process of cell *apoptosis*(death) in cancer of the prostate. This process of cell destruction is seen no more when the cancer becomes hormone resistant.

Q. What is the survival rate with Hormone Therapy?

Hormone Therapy is not expected to **completely** eradicate prostate cancer. Prostate cancer has a mixture of cells; some are hormone-sensitive and some are hormone-insensitive. As the disease advances, the population of hormone-insensitive cells increases, and the beneficial effects of hormone treatment decrease.

Although a tumor may apparently disappear, **microscopic cancer** persists. Despite treatment, 50% of the patients who receive Hormone Therapy live for only 2-3 years. On the average, progression of the disease becomes evident 12-18 months after hormone treatment. Once a relapse occurs, the prognosis is very poor; the six-month survival rate for such cases is 50%.

LASER SURGERY

Q. Will you talk about Laser Surgery?

Certainly! Laser Surgery can also be used in cases of **localized prostate cancer** in place of a Radical Prostatectomy or radiation treatment, or in patients who have failed radiation treatment. A laser penetrates the cancer tissue and **destroys it with heat**. This procedure is carried out through a *cystoscope* placed in the *urethra*.

Once located at the prostate, the laser beam is fired which precisely burns away the cancer. Laser Surgery is much simpler than Radical Prostatectomy; the hospital stay is short (usually overnight) and recovery is fast. This is a fairly new treatment, and as yet, clinical experience with laser surgery for prostate cancer is insufficient to evaluate its efficacy.

CRYOSURGERY

Cryosurgery (cryoablation or *cryotherapy)* is the **destruction of cancer cells by freezing**. This method of treatment has been in use since the 1960's. With the continual improvement in equipment and technique and the use of ultrasound technology *Cryosurgery* is now a precise, rapid and efficient treatment.

Q. When is Cryosurgery used?

Patients with localized prostate cancer who are **unable to tolerate** surgery of Radical Prostatectomy, or in place of, or in addition to Radiation Therapy when the latter has failed.

Q. What is involved in Cryosurgery?

Cryosurgery is carried out under general anesthesia or under a spinal anesthesia (where only the lower body is anesthetized). Under ultrasound guidance, *cryoprobes* (usually 5) are passed through the skin behind the *scrotum* and precisely positioned in the prostate. Liquid nitrogen (at -180°C to -190°C) is then introduced into the prostate through the probes. A catheter tube is placed in the bladder through an opening made above the pubic area, and warm water (40°C) is circulated continually to protect the *urethra* during the freezing process.

Cryosurgery requires a short hospital stay of about two days. A catheter remains in the bladder for one to three weeks after surgery or until the patient can fully recover normal urination.

Q. What are the possible complications?

The major risk is that of impotence, which is 50% to 65%. Incontinence is reported in the 3% to 4% range. Other complications which occur less commonly includes a puncture between the *urethra* and *rectum,* a narrowing of the *bladder neck* caused by scarring, and a narrowing of the *urethral*, also caused by scarring. These can all be corrected with surgery.

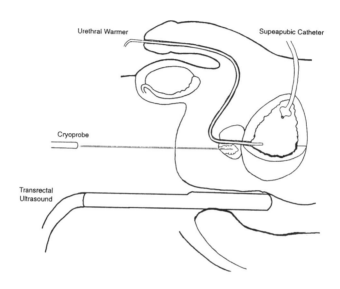

Cryosurgery

Q. Can Cryosurgery be considered a cure?

After *Cryosurgery*, the PSA of the patient is checked periodically every 6-12 weeks to monitor the complete elimination of the cancer. A biopsy is done after 3 months as a further check. If any residual cancer is suspected, *Cryosurgery* can be repeated.

Recent biopsy reports have shown encouraging results. Residual cancer has been found in up to 20% of the cases treated only once; the second treatment is able to lower the rate of residual cancer to 5%.

Q. What are the advantages of Microwave Heat Therapy?

It's called *Hyperthermia Therapy,* a procedure which uses heat over 45°C (77°F) to kill cancerous cells. In this treatment for prostate cancer, microwaves are used as a heat source and introduced into the prostate through a rectal probe; the *rectum* is cooled to protect it from damage.

Like *Cryosurgery, Hyperthermia Therapy* is used in cases of localized cancer in place of Radical Prostatectomy or Radiation Therapy, or when Radiation Therapy has failed.

At the present time, *Hyperthermia Therapy* is rarely used because clinical experience is not yet available to evaluate the benefits or complications of this treatment. It is possible that Hyperthermia Therapy may develop into a useful treatment.

CHEMOTHERAPY

Q. When is Chemotherapy used?

For patients with **advanced** prostate cancer, the choice of treatment is very limited, and about 20% to 30% of the patients diagnosed do not respond to hormone treatments. Of those who do, half will become desensitized to the treatment within one year. Chemotherapy is then used, not so much to prolong survival as to relieve the symptoms of metastastic (spreading) cancer.

This treatment is not without the risk of possible severe toxic side-effects. However, the risks must be weighed against the possibility of relief on an individual basis.

Q. What is involved in Chemotherapy?

In general, conventional anticancer drugs have not been as effective in prostate cancer as in some other cancers. Different drugs have been used alone and in combination, but there is no standard regimen for Hormone Resistant Prostate Cancer. Some of the drugs which have been reported to give encouraging responses are:

- *Estamustine®*
- *Vinblastine®*
- *Etopside®*
- *Doxorubicin®*

Q. What results can be expected from Chemotherapy?

It varies with the extent of the disease, general condition of the patient, and the anticancer drug used. On the average, relief from the pain and symptoms of advanced cancer last for only six months.

Q. Talk about Pain Management.

Pain usually occurs late in the disease, arising from the metastastic deposits of cancer in the bones. When the pain is comparatively mild, it can be controlled by non-narcotic medications such as *Tylenol* and *Ibuprofens*. In more severe pain, narcotic medications such as *codeine, demerol* and *morphine* may have to be used.

Pain can be very persistent in some cases and may severely deteriorate the quality of life. In such cases pain medications can be given through a special infusion pump implanted in the body which constantly delivers medication for several months at a time. Recently, pain management has made huge advances, and different methods are available to control pain effectively.

Q. How about Localized External Radiation Therapy?

External Beam Radiation to a localized area of bone causing pain is very effective in relieving pain. Improvement can start within 48 hours of radiation treatment. Good relief of pain has been found in about 80% of the patients.

However, pain is not always located in a single bone site. If the pain is originating from several sites, radiation can be given to a wide area (*Hemibody Radiation*) but this involves risk of toxic effects on the bone marrow.

Bone marrow ceases manufacturing blood cells and platelets; this caused *anemia,* low resistance to infections, and a high tendency to bleed.

Q. What is Strontium-89?

This was explained earlier when we talked about treatment of prostate cancer; it can also serve to control pain. *Strontium-89* is a **radioactive isotope** which has been used with good results in relieving pain from the spreading (*metastastic*) deposits of cancer in the bones. It is given as an intravenous injection.

After settling in the cancerous bones, it emits radiation into the cancer as an **Internal Radiation Therapy**. It has been used alone or in combination with external radiation or *Chemotherapy* to enhance its effect. It has been reported to give pain relief in up to 80% of the patients with *metastastic* cancer in the bones.

Author's Note:
Some of the surgery and treatments for cancer are repeated several times in this book—for two reasons. One, is because the various treatments are good for special types of prostate cancer only, yet on other types, they are used in **conjunction** *with specific methods.*

Two, I'd like all men to realize how dangerous and troublesome (if not lethal) prostate cancer can be to either you, a brother, father or close friend or relative. After reading my book, I'm hoping you'll get a yearly prostate exam and encourage each of them to do likewise.

Part 5

Treatment Selection

If you are concerned about prostate cancer or have been diagnosed with it, chances are you have read every page in this book. You know about **Hormone Therapy** and **Radical Prostatectomy**, and you don't have long to make up your mind to be tested or to have an operation. So now comes the selection of treatment.

Of course, other than this book, you must talk with your urologist and have him/her explain each operation in detail. Together—academically—select a treatment. You see, after the diagnosis of prostate cancer is made, the next question is to see **which would be the best treatment for it!** There are different options available. Each has its own advantages and drawbacks. The decision is not a simple matter.

However, there are several factors to influence your choice of treatment. For instance . . .

> Your Age
> Your General Health
> The Stage of Cancer (*extent of cancer*)
> The Grade of Cancer (*aggressiveness*)
> PSA

Of these, the most important is the stage or the extent of cancer. To help you make this treatment selection, your urologist will explain that the extent of the cancer is paramount. It is divided into three categories:

✔Cancer confined to the prostate.
✔Cancer with limited local extension outside the prostate.
✔Cancer that has spread to lymph nodes and distant organs.

CANCER CONFINED TO THE PROSTATE

Stage A_1 Cancer (T_{1a})
Treatment Options . . . .
                    Watchful Waiting
                    Radical Retropubic Prostectomy

As stated earlier, it is not possible to detect Stage A_1 Cancer solely from a Digital Rectal Examination (DRE); it must be diagnosed when prostate tissue is removed (by TURP or Trans-Urethral Resection of the Prostate) to relieve obstruction in presumably a benign enlarged prostate and 5% or less of the tissue removed shows cancer.

In 15% of such cases, a repeat TURP would show no more cancer. In spite of this, there is no certainty that the remaining prostate has no cancer. But, *generally Stage A_1 Cancer is not an aggressive tumor.* This is borne out in a study of 148 patients, by a Veterans Administration Cooperative Urological Research Group, where only 6.8% showed any progression of the disease.

In yet another study it was estimated that on the average, it takes 17.5 years for stage A_1 cancer to show progression. This shows a potentially slow growing cancer and therefore aggressive treatment is not always warranted. This type of cancer can be watched and aggressive treatment can be held off unless signs of progression appear.

Now, this is when age becomes a factor. For those in their fifties, since the expected life span is long enough for the cancer to progress to become life threatening, an aggressive approach using **Radical Prostatectomy** would be advisable. It has been proven that 20% of these Stage 1 Cancers are actually more extensive than initially believed and would have progressed faster than expected.

Stage A_2 (T_{1b}) Cancer and Stage B(T_2)
Treatment Options . . . .
        Radical Retropubic Prostatectomy
        Radiation Therapy
        Watchful Waiting
        Cryosurgery

If you have been diagnosed as having a Stage A_2 Cancer, you're aware that it is not possible to detect this stage by a Digital Rectal Examination only; like A_1 Cancer, it is diagnosed unexpectedly when prostate tissue is removed to relieve obstruction in presumably benign enlargement of the prostate.

Unlike Stage A_1 Cancer, Stage A_2 Cancer has a potentially serious prognosis. **Progression** is found in 35% of the A_2 Cancers, and Lymph Node metastasis is found in 25%.

The average time of progression of this Stage A_2 cancer is 4.75 years as compared to 17.5 years in Stage A_1. Therefore, this cancer demands **aggressive** treatment similar to that recommended for Stage **B** Cancer.

Stage **B** Cancer can be detected by Digital Rectal Examination. This cancer is confined within the prostate and is therefore potentially curable, and aggressive treatment like surgery or Radiation Therapy is generally recommended.

Radical Prostatectomy is the most ideal treatment for localized cancer of the prostate. This can cure you if the cancer is confined solely in the prostate. However, clinical estimation of the extent (or stage) of cancer is not always reliable; 40-60% of the cancers **clinically presumed** to be confined within the prostate, at operation, are found to have penetrated beyond the capsule of the prostate!

Most of these cancers cannot be removed without leaving some margins of cancer behind, and surgery cannot be considered curative. The residual cancer will eventually grow locally or spread.

The prognosis is adversely affected with residual cancer after surgery. Survival rates in patients who had incomplete removal of cancer reduces to 50% as compared to those who had no residual cancer after surgery. Further treatment is generally recommended if there is residual cancer after surgery.

Recent studies show that patients with residual cancer are benefitted by **Postoperative Radiation Therapy**. Some patients with minimal microscopic residual cancer may be watched for evidence of the disease progression before further treatment is given, but control of the disease is better when the residual cancer is treated early, rather than leave it unattended to allow it to grow to a large size.

Surgery has the best results when the cancer is completely removed. In such patients, PSA comes down to an undetectable level. Survival is similar to that expected in normal people in that age group. In terms of **recurrence of cancer,** surgery is superior to any other treatment, when survival and free of disease is considered.

RADICAL PROSTATECTOMY

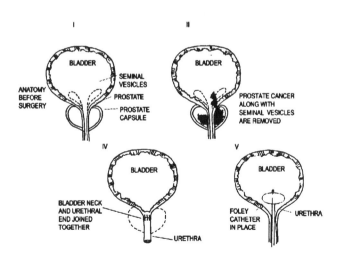

A study of 3,170 patients, with clinically localized cancer who underwent Radical Prostatectomy at the *Mayo Clinic*, reported that 10 and 15-year disease-specific-survival was 90% and 82%.

Surgery is considered the "gold standard" in the treatment of **organ-confined cancer** of the prostate. Surgery, of course, is not without the risk of some potential complications. Of these, the most important complications are **sexual impotence** and **incontinence** of urine. Risk of impotence is quite high, occurring in 30-70% of patients after surgery. It is more likely to occur in older patients. It is also more frequent in patients who have more extensive cancer.

Smaller cancers can be removed with less risk of injury to the potency nerves. Some older patients may be impotent even before the diagnosis of cancer of the prostate is made. To such patients, this complication of surgery would not matter. Patients who develop permanent impotence can be greatly improved with different methods available for treatment. It is of such importance that the next chapter tells most of what you would like to know and, happily, all positive.

Incontinence of urine occurs much less frequently than impotence; 95% of the patients have full control of urination after surgery. Those who do develop incontinence can be treated with medications, collagen injections in the *bladder neck* or implantation of an artificial *sphincter,* depending upon the severity of the condition.

Radiation Therapy has undergone a large degree of progress and refinement in the equipment and techniques of radiotherapy. These have increased the efficacy and reduced the potential complications of this treatment. An extensive study of literature showed that in clinically localized cancer, 10-year disease-specific-survival for **Radiation Therapy** was 74% as compared to 93% for **Radical Prostatectomy.** That makes the odds in your favor by more than 9 to 1!

Some studies have shown even better results in favor of surgery. In comparing results of Radiation Therapy and surgery, one has to keep in mind that there may be some bias in selection of more favorable cases for surgery.

Be cognizant of the fact that the results of Radiation Therapy depend greatly on the extent (stage) of the cancer. Survival rates are better when the treatment is given in the earlier stages than in the more advanced disease. In a series of 1,119 cases of Stage **A** Cancer, 15-year survival, after radiation therapy, matched the normal life expectancy, and in Stage **B** Cancer, it was 5% short of that.

In treatment of cancer confined to the prostate, surgery has an excellent chance of **removing the disease completely!** In contrast, chances of finding residual cancer on a needle biopsy after radiation therapy are 25 to 55%, again, depending upon the stage of the cancer.

However, significance of residual cancer on a needle biopsy is not quite clear. Some people argue that the residual cancer seen after radiation does not have the same capability to grow and spread as the cancer before radiation treatment. On the other hand, several reports have shown that local recurrence and distant spread is more common in patients who show cancer on the biopsy after Radiation Therapy than those who show no residual cancer.

Radiation Therapy is a much less aggressive treatment than surgery and has fewer complications. It can be tolerated more easily by the patients who may not withstand surgery because of poor general health.

Now, let's talk more about **Watchful Waiting,** Since prostate cancer is a slow-growing tumor, and Watchful Waiting is a reasonable alternative treatment in **selected cases of localized cancer of the prostate** (advanced age and poor physical condition mostly).

In a pooled analysis of 828 patients with localized cancer of the prostate who were managed with Watchful Waiting, it was estimated that the patients had 8 to 10% higher risk of dying at 10 years as compared to those treated with aggressive treatment like Radiation Therapy or surgery.

It appeared that with follow-up for longer than 10 years, the outcome of Watchful Waiting could lag further when compared with aggressive treatment. In some reports 5 and 10-year cancer-specific-survival has been shown to be almost similar to that with aggressive treatment.

In men who have a **short life expectancy** because of advanced age or ill health due to other ailments, Watchful Waiting would be a suitable method of cancer management. Such men would not be able to realize the long-term advantage of aggressive treatment and could be saved the risk of possible complications associated with surgery or Radiation Therapy.

On the other hand, Watchful Waiting would not be advisable for a younger man with localized cancer of the prostate which could be treated for a cure with aggressive treatment because of the long life expectancy. Too, the young man is usually much stronger and can tolerate an aggressive treatment. And if there are complications, these too can be treated.

Cryosurgery (destruction of cancer with freezing temperature) can be used to treat **localized cancer confined to the prostate**. It is a comparatively newer technique and enough long term results are not available yet to evaluate the efficacy of this treatment. Recent reports, however, have shown encouraging results. Re-biopsy of the prostate, 3 months after *Cryotherapy*, has shown residual cancer in 5 to 20% of the patients. After repeating the treatment, the rate of residual cancer has been even less.

Cryosurgery is a much simpler procedure than surgery, although it is not a completely risk-free treatment; it has a high risk of causing impotence! Other potential complications include incontinence, or injury to the rectum or the bladder. So far, *Cryosurgery* is performed in limited centers in this country and most urologists have not yet started using this treatment.

CANCER WITH LIMITED LOCAL EXTENSION

Stage C (T$_3$) Cancer
Treatment Options . . . .
        Radiation Therapy
        Hormone Therapy plus Radiation Therapy
        Surgery plus Hormone Therapy
        Cryosurgery

With cancer that is outside the prostate that has penetrated through the capsule of the prostate or extended into the seminal vesicle, it is classified as Stage **C** (Stage **T$_3$** according to the Int'l Classification). **Radiation Therapy** is the best choice for this cancer.

External Beam Radiation can cover a wide field, including the prostate and its surrounding area where cancer in Stage **C** extends. Effectiveness of Radiation Therapy is improved with newer techniques using *Conformal Therapy.*

A combination of **external beam radiation** and **local irradiation** with implantation of radioactive material in the prostate (*brachytherapy*) can deliver higher dosages without increasing the risk of damage to the surrounding normal tissues.

However, the results of Radiation Therapy in Stage C cancer are not expected to be as good as in the early stages when cancer is confined to the prostate (Stage **A** and Stage **B**). Average survival after Radiation Therapy in Stage **A** Cancer is almost similar to the normal life expectancy. In Stage **B** Cancer, it is within 16% of the normal, but in Stage **C**, it is 26% below normal expected.

Hormone Therapy has limited benefit in Stage **C** cancer, according to a Veterans Administration Cooperative Urological Research Group study, which showed that Hormone Therapy slowed progression of Stage **C** cancer but it did not result in prolongation of life.

Stage **C** Cancer has high likelihood of distant spread and local treatment alone has high chances of failure. However, a combination of local treatment with hormone treatment has been more promising. *Hormone treatment has been used in combination with radiation therapy with better results than any single treatment alone!*

The National Cancer Institute of Canada is conducting a randomized clinical trial to Compare Hormone Therapy alone, versus Hormone Therapy and Radiation Therapy for Stage **C** Cancer. Results of this study will greatly help in selecting treatment for Stage **C** Cancer.

Surgery is generally not recommended in Stage **C** Cancer because the disease has extended beyond the capsule of the prostate making complete removal of cancer not feasible. However, some reports have shown good results when Radical Prostatectomy is combined with Hormone Therapy. Hormone Therapy is often used before surgery (*neoadjuvent therapy*) to reduce the size of Stage **C** Cancer.

Cryosurgery has also been used in Stage **C** Cancer, however, sufficient experience is not available to asses the outcome.

CANCER WITH SPREAD

Stage D_1 Cancer
Treatment Options . . . .
> Surgery and Hormone Therapy
> Radiation and Hormone Therapy
> Hormone Therapy

Stage D_1 is when spread in the pelvic lymph nodes is minimal, showing small microscopic deposits or when only a single lymph node is involved, some reports have shown good results with Radical Prostate Surgery and immediate Hormone Therapy rather than Hormone Therapy alone.

Statistics show a 10-year disease-specific survival rates in Stage D_1 Cancer treated with different methods were as follows.

Surgery and Hormone therapy	78%
Radiation and Hormone therapy	66%
Hormone therapy alone	39%

Stage D_2 Cancer
Treatment Options . . . .
> Hormone Therapy
> LHRH Analogs
> Orchiectomy
> Antiandrogens
> Second Line Hormone Agents

Hormone Therapy is the standard treatment when

cancer has spread to Lymph Nodes, or to the bones and other organs Stage D_2. Early Hormone Therapy, instituted as soon as diagnosis of *metastastic* cancer is made, gives better suppression of disease and better survival than delayed treatment.

Hormone therapy is most active in early stages when cancer is still hormone-sensitive. In later stages, cancer gradually becomes hormone **resistant!**

Urologists also use what are called *second line hormonal agents* when Metastatic Prostate Cancer becomes hormone resistant so that the usual hormone therapy becomes ineffective (Stage D_3). At this stage, second line hormonal agents such as *Ketoconazol* and *Prednisone* are used with some relief.

Chemotherapy is also used in hormone resistant cancer with often good remissions.

Maximal Androgen Blockade is achieved when male hormones are blocked from both sources, namely the *testes* and the adrenal glands. The *testes* can either be removed surgically or suppressed completely by using LHRH analog drugs such as *Lupron*® or *Zoladex*® . Androgens from the adrenals can be suppressed by antiandrogen drugs like *Flutamide, Bicalutamide* or *Nilutamide.*

Although 95% of the androgens in the body are produced by the *testes,* the small contribution of androgen production by the adrenals is also important in cancer of the prostate. Literature is in favor of maximal **androgen blockades** which gives significantly better cancer-specific-survival than surgical removal of the *testes (orchiectomy)* or suppression of the *testes* with LHRH drugs.

Case History

One of my patients had TURP (*Transurethral Resection of Prostate*) 7 years ago when he was 72-years old. Clinically he was diagnosed to have a benign enlargement of the prostate. Only part of the prostate tissue was removed (TURP) to relieve obstruction to urine flow. On pathological examination, all the tissue removed was benign except for a single chip which showed a focus of cancer. The cancer was well differentiated low grade type. His PSA was normal.

It appeared that this minute, low grade Stage A_1 cancer would not grow large enough to cause a problem during the patient's lifetime. As per my recommendation, and with his consent, it was decided to manage this patient on Watchful Waiting. Periodic Digital Rectal Examination and checking of PSA level were carried out.

During this time he has not shown any abnormality and has also remained symptom free. He is now 79-years old and his chances are good of having no threat to life from the prostate cancer. He has been saved from surgery or any form of **aggressive treatment** and its possible complications so far, and most likely the rest of his life.

HOPE THROUGH RESEARCH

Research scientists and surgeons are busy in their laboratories working on methods of prevention and cure of all sorts of cancer. More progress has been made in medicine during these past two decades than in the history of the world and some day soon there WILL be a discovery to rid us of this dreaded malady.

Chemoprevention

One of the methods recently introduced is a hormonal agent *Finasteride,* considered likely to have a possible role in **preventing prostate cancer**. It is normally used in the treatment of benign enlargement of the prostate where it decreases the size of the prostate and reduces the PSA level.

The National Cancer Institute and other oncology groups have sponsored a clinical trial and will enroll 18,000 men who will be given *Finasteride* or placebo and they will be monitored for 7-10 years. This study will eventually show if prostate cancer can be prevented with this hormonal agent.

Antibodies

Some antibodies have been developed but they are more specific to the prostate than prostate cancer. It would be most desirable to have antibodies which would specifically *destroy prostate cancer cells.* Even destruction of the whole prostate gland with antibodies would be an advantage because the prostate has no useful function other than helping in fertility.

Gene Therapy

Genetic research has made great advances in the biology of cancer. Several genes have been found which promote growth and spread of different cancers. These genes are called **oncogenes.** Although no gene has been specifically associated with causation of prostate cancer, involvement of genes has been recognized in the advanced cancers of the prostate.

Genes that inhibit the growth and progress of cancer are called *suppressor genes* or *anti-cancer genes.* Loss of these anti-cancer genes has been associated with cancer of the prostate.

With present technology, it is possible to replace an abnormal gene or add a gene to a cell. In this way the beneficial effect of an anti-cancer gene can be restored. Gene Therapy has already shown promising results in some cancers. In the future, a cancer vaccine may become possible to protect against prostate cancer.

Part 6

Impotence Relief After Surgery

Impotence occurs in 30%-70% of the cases following Radical Prostatectomy. In spite of the modern surgical techniques, it is not always possible to save the nerves. The younger you are, the more likely it is that you will recover full sexual function. If the tumor is localized to the prostate, your surgeon will use **surgical techniques** which save the nerves on both sides of the prostate and increase the chances of full recovery of potency.

Even if the nerves can be saved on just one side, chances of recovery remain good. In bulky tumors, or when the cancer has spread beyond the capsule surrounding the prostate, nerve saving is not always possible; in these cases it is more prudent to make sure all the cancer is removed.

Regardless of the outcome, there are now means to help you enjoy a satisfying sexual life after such an operation. In cases where a full recovery is expected, return of potency may take six months or more. During this time, your doctor may recommend one of the following treatments to aid in sexual rehabilitation:

PENILE INJECTION

There are three drugs available that can be injected

into the tissue of the penis which produce erection. This erection lasts for 30-60 minutes. If it lasts as long as 3-4 hours, you may develop *priapism* which must be reversed by your physician using counteracting drugs, also by injection.

Case History

Dr. X is a 58-year-old physician colleague of mine. He had Radical Retropubic Prostatectomy two years ago, with only partial recovery of sexual function but his erection was not strong enough for a satisfactory intercourse. He told me that he and his wife had accepted the circumstances and were quite contented. I suggested a vacuum device or penile injection. He decided to use injection therapy. I gave him the first injection of *prostaglandin E_1*. He has been using the injections successfully—and regularly!

URETHRAL SUPPOSITORIES

These suppositories are inserted into the urethra (urinary channel of the penis). The medication is absorbed into the tissue and this produces an erection for 30+ minutes. The photo, furnished by Vivus Inc., shows a Transurethral System (Muse®) that introduces a small pellet which contains *alprostadil.*

VACUUM ERECTION DEVICES

In this method, the penis is placed in a cylinder in which a vacuum is created to bring blood flow to the penis. Once an erection is attained, it is maintained up to 30 minutes with a rubber tension ring around the base of the penis. One device shown is a **mechanical** hand pump. The other is **battery operated**. Your urologist will have videos and/or the device itself to show you. Vacuum erection devices have been used with good results by many patients.

Photo courtesy of Vivus, Inc.

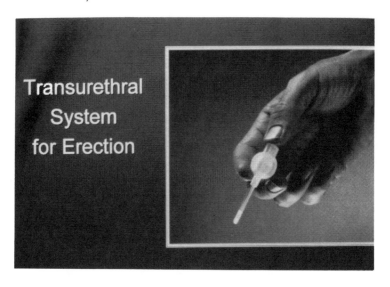

Transurethral Suppository System

Case History

Mr. Z, was not able to have an erection after his prostate surgery. Different options of treatment were discussed with him. He liked the idea of the vacuum pump. He went ahead and bought the device and since then has been very pleased with it. He told me that this was the best investment he had ever made.

Photo furnished by Osbon Medical Systems

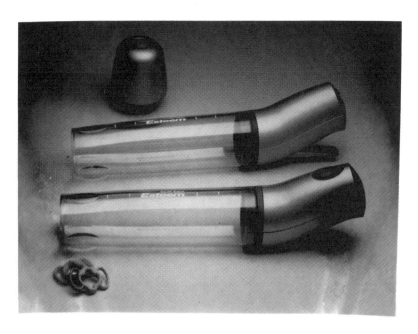

*Mechanical and Battery Operated
Vacuum Erection Devices*

Impotence is not permanent in every man after Radical Prostate Surgery; one third or more recover sexual potency! The wife of an executive who underwent Radical Prostate Surgery a year ago, accidently met me in the hospital and could not resist shouting to me, "He did it! He did it!" She then explained to me that it took him a year to gradually recover his sexual function and the last few times it was just like normal. I was very pleased to hear that because he was comparatively young (late fifties) and was depressed because of sexual difficulties.

In some cases, if the erection is not rigid enough, the vacuum device can be used in conjunction with the injection. The main complication of these medications is the possibility of a persistent erection, a condition called *priapism*. If the erection does not subside after 2-3 hours, a physician should be contacted. This can be a very uncomfortable condition but can be treated with an injection of medication to reverse the erection.

PENILE PROSTHESIS

Some patients who prefer not to use vacuum erection devices or penile injections, a *penile prosthesis* is more suitable for them. However, since this method involves surgery and is permanent, I advise that the decision to implant a prosthesis be postponed until it is certain that no recovery of normal potency is expected.

Prosthetics come in two main types: inflatable and semi-rigid. The **inflatable type** keeps the penis soft until an erection is desired. A pump then induces an erection in the penis. This is by far the most successful but the cost, $10,000+ limits the number of patients who can afford it.

The semi-rigid type is not collapsible but can be bent for concealment, and since this latter type of prosthesis does not have a pump system, there is less risk of mechanical failure. Again, your urologist will have more pertinent information for you.

Photo courtesy of American Medical System

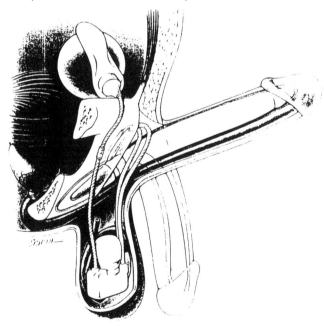

Inflatable Penile Prosthesis

Case History

A patient of mine is a professional *mariachi* singer. Impotence was a great deficiency in his otherwise very high profile and happy life. He selected to have a semirigid penile prosthesis. The prosthesis has given him the sense of fulfillment. He tells me that if I ever decide to give a big party, he would bring his whole mariachi band to performance free for me. He said, "Doc, you made me happy. I want to make you happy at your party."

Case History

Mr. Y, wanted to have a **semi-rigid** penile prosthesis. I put the prosthesis in him 3 years ago. I was surprised to hear that he has never used it. I asked him why he wanted the prosthesis if he was not going to use it? He said, he was divorced and had no sexual partner but he was still happy that he had the prosthesis. It gave him a sense of adequacy and security.

Complete recovery of normal sexual function varies with each patient. Even without the recovery of erection and without the semen, most patients can experience orgasm. If recovery is not complete, some forms of therapy such as the ones above are an answer.

The subject of a penile prosthesis is a vast area to discuss and those who are interested need to talk at length with their urologist, who can show them films, photos and case histories of those who have undergone this type of surgery.

Photo courtesy of American Medical System

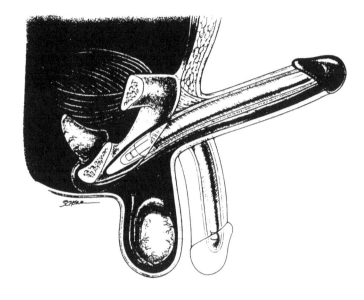

Semi-Rigid Penile Prosthesis

GLOSSARY

ACINI: Small pockets lined with cells.

ADVANCED CANCER: Cancer that has spread outside the prostate.

AGE-ADJUSTED PSA: Variation of normal PSA, according to the age of the person.

AGGRESSIVE TREATMENT: Surgery or radiation therapies are called aggressive because of the possibility of potential complications.

ANEMIA: Inadequate blood.

ANESTHESIA: Method of controlling pain and sensation during surgical procedure.

ANEUPLOID: Abnormal DNA content representing different number of chromosomes.

ANTIANDROGENS: Drugs which inhibit the action of testosterone on prostate cancer.

ARTIFICIAL SPHINCTER: An inflatable cuff that is placed around the urethra. Inflation of this circular balloon closes the urethra to prevent leakage when urination is not desired.

BENIGN ENLARGEMENT OF PROSTATE: Enlargement of the prostate without cancer. It occurs commonly in middle aged and older men.

BIOPSY: A specimen removed from the tissue for microscopic examination.

BLADDER: An organ in the pelvis for storage of urine.

BONE SCAN: Picture of the skeleton taken after intravenous administration of nuclear material. Cancer deposits in the bones show abnormally high uptake of the nuclear material.

CANCER: Abnormal growth of cells which can spread in the body and eventually become lethal.

CAT SCAN: Computer Assisted Tomography Scan—gives X-ray images in more than one dimensional view.

CATHETER: A tube used to drain the urine.

CELL: The basic component of an organ or tissue.

CHEMISTRY PROFILE: A group of tests for routine evaluation of blood chemistry.

CHEMOPREVENTION: Medication to prevent cancer.

CHEMOTHERAPY:Treatment of cancer with drugs which destroy cancer cells.

CHROMOSOMES: Nuclear material of the cell containing genetic material.

CLINICALLY INSIGNIFICANT CANCER: Cancer that does not grow enough during the lifetime of the patient to cause any ill effect on health.

CLINICALLY SIGNIFICANT CANCER: Cancer that grows to cause symptoms and eventually death.

COMA: State of unconsciousness.

CRYOPROBES: Cooling probes used in cryosurgery.

CRYOSURGERY: Also called cryoablation (or cryotherapy). Freezing the prostate to destroy the cancer cells.

DIETHYLSTILBESTROL (DES): A female hormone used in the treatment of advanced cancer of the prostate.

DIGITAL RECTAL EXAMINATION: Examination of the prostate performed with a finger through the rectum.

DIPLOID: Normal DNA content representing two sets of chromosomes.

DNA: (Deoxyribonucleic Acid) Chemical ingredient that makes the nucleus of a cell.

EARLY STAGE CANCER: Cancer that is still confined to the prostate and can be treated to achieve a cure.

ESTROGEN: A female hormone used in the treatment of advanced cancer of the prostate.

FREE PSA: In the blood, PSA exists in a free form and in a form in which it is bound with other components of blood. The sum of the Free and the Bound PSA is the total PSA.

FROZEN SECTION: Technique of freezing biopsy tissue to form ice cubes to facilitate cutting into microscopic slices for examination.

GENERAL ANESTHESIA: Deep sleep is induced so that pain and sensations are completely lost.

GENETIC: Related to inheritance through genes.

GONADOTROPIC HORMONE: Two Luteinizing hormones (LH) and Follicle Stimulating Hormone (FSH) are secreted by the pituitary and stimulate the testes to produce testosterone (male hormone produced in the testes) and sperm.

GRADES OF CANCER: Some cancers are potentially more aggressive than the others. Degree of aggressiveness is assessed on microscopic examination of the cancer. Potential aggressiveness is classified in grades of tumor.

GYNECOMASTIA: Enlargement of breasts. This can occur in men receiving estrogens for the treatment of advanced cancer of the prostate.

HEMATURIA: Blood in the urine.

HESITANCY: Urination does not start immediately when desired.

HORMONE-INSENSITIVE: Cancer which shows no response to hormone therapy.

HORMONE SENSITIVE: Cancers that respond to hormone treatment.

HORMONE THERAPY: Use of hormones to treat the cancer.

HOT FLASHES: The body suddenly feels hot and sweaty. Hot flashes occur in women during menopause. Hot flashes can occur as a side effect of LHRH hormone therapy for advanced cancer of the prostate.

HYPERTHERMIA THERAPY: Treatment of cancer with destruction of cancer cells by the use of high heat produced by microwaves.

HYPOTHALAMUS: Part of the brain that produces (LHRH) to stimulate the pituitary.

IMPOTENCE: Inability to achieve erection of the penis.

INCONTINENCE: Loss of urine without control.

INVASION: Penetration into surrounding structure. Cancer has the potential of invasion into surrounding tissues beyond its normal boundaries.

LASER SURGERY: A laser is used through the cystoscope to destroy prostate cancer.

LATENT CANCER: Cancer that causes no ill effect and is only found unexpectedly at a postmortem for death due to some unrelated cause.

LHRH:(Luteinizing hormone releasing hormones). A hormone that is produced in the base of the brain and stimulates the pituitary to secrete its luteinizing hormone (LH), which stimulates the testes to produce the male hormone—testosterone.

LIBIDO: Sex drive.

LOCALIZED PROSTATE CANCER: A cancer that is confined to the prostate and has not spread anywhere else in the body.

LUPRON (TAP Pharmaceutical): Synthetic LHRH, used in the treatment of advanced cancer of the prostate.

LYMPH NODES: Small structures varying from a few millimeters to a centimeter into which lymphatic vessels drain lymphatic fluid. Lymph nodes trap bacteria and cancer cells and try to destroy them.

LYMPHATIC SYSTEM: System of lymph nodes and the lymphatic vessels.

LYMPHOCELE: A collection of fluid leaking from the lymphatics.

MAGNETIC RESONANCE IMAGING: (MRI) Images of the body taken by modern technique of resonance instead of X-rays.

MALIGNANT: Abnormal growth of cells which spread in the body and eventually become lethal.

METASTASIS: Distant spread of cancer.

NEUROVASCULAR BUNDLE: A collection of nerves and blood vessels which lie behind and on the side of the prostate. These nerves are responsible for erection of the penis.

NUCLEUS: A central part of a cell comprised of a collection of chromosomes.

ORCHIECTOMY: Surgical removal of the testes employed in the treatment of advanced cancer of the prostate.

"PELVIC" NODE LAPAROSCOPIC DISSECTION: Removal of pelvic lymph nodes through tiny incisions through which scopes and instruments are inserted for visualization and dissection.

PENILE INJECTIONS FOR IMPOTENCE: Medications injected into the body of the penis to cause erection.

PENILE PROSTHESIS: Prosthesis surgically implanted in the penis to achieve erection. Prosthesis can be semi-rigid or inflatable. The latter has a balloon which can be pumped when erection is desired.

PERINEAL PROSTATECTOMY: Surgical technique that uses incision through the perineal area to remove the prostate.

PITUITARY GLAND: A pea-size gland situated in the base of the skull. Besides other hormones it produces the luteinizing hormone which stimulates the testes to produce testosterone.

PLACEBO: A blank pill with no active medicine in it.

PRIAPISM: Persistent erection that would not subside.

PROSTATE: A male reproductive organ, situated below the urinary bladder. It produces fluid to transport the sperm. In men of advanced age, the prostate enlarges and may obstruct urine flow. It is the site of this commonest cancer of man.

PROSTATIC ACID PHOSPHATASE: Acid phosphatase is pro-duced by the prostate and released in the blood in circulation. High values of prostatic acid phosphatase may indicate the presence of cancer.

PROSTATIC INTRAEPITHELIAL NEOPLASIA:(PIN) Malignancy is limited to the cells on the surface of the glands without evidence of invasion of the deeper tissues.

PSA: Prostate Specific Antigen. A substance produced exclusively from the prostate. High value of PSA in the blood is due to the large size of the prostate, inflammation, or cancer of the prostate.

PSA DENSITY: PSA value per cc volume of the prostate.

PSA VELOCITY:The rate of change of PSA over a period of time.

RADIATION THERAPY: Treatment of cancer by using radiation to destroy the cancer cells.

RADICAL PROSTATECTOMY:Total removal of the prostate along with seminal vesicles.

RECTUM:The lowest part of the intestinal tract.

REGIONAL ANESTHESIA: Spinal or epidural anesthesia produce loss of sensation and pain in the region of surgery and do not generate the effect of deep sleep.

RETENTION OF URINE: Inability to urinate causing accumulation of urine in the bladder.

RETROPUBIC PROSTATECTOMY: Surgical technique that uses incision through the lower part of the abdomen to remove the prostate.

SALVAGE SURGERY: Surgery to remove the prostate after radiation or cryosurgery has failed.

SCREENING: Examining healthy men to detect prostate cancer. Screening usually involves digital rectal examination (DRE) and blood test to check the level of Prostate Specific Antigen (PSA).

SEMEN: Fluid containing prostatic secretions and sperms.

SPHINCTER: A group of muscle fibers which surround the urethra and shut off urine when urination is not desired.

SPINAL CORD: A long cord composed of nerve tissue that connects the brain with nerves in the body.

SPINAL AND EPIDURAL ANESTHETIC: Method of anesthesia in which medication is injected in or around the spinal cord to numb the body without inducing sleep.

STAGES OF CANCER: The size and the extent of cancer classified into groups.

TESTES: Part of the male reproductive organ. They produce sperm and the male hormone, testosterone.

TESTOSTERONE: Male hormone, mainly produced in the testes.

TETRAPLOID: Abnormal DNA content representing 4 sets of chromosomes.

TISSUE: A collection of cells.

ULTRASOUND EXAMINATION: Picture of the prostate generated by ultrasound echoes to detect presence of cancer.

ULTRASOUND TRANSDUCER: Instrument that transmits and receives echoes.

UREMIA: Accumulation of toxic waste products of the body.

URETER: A tube that allows the urine to pass from the kidney to the urinary bladder.

URETHRA: Urinary channel below the bladder to evacuate urine.

URGENCY IN URINATION: Sudden, strong desire to urinate.

URINALYSIS: A group of tests for routine evaluation of the urine.

VACUUM ERECTION DEVICE: A device to achieve erection using vacuum to draw blood into the penis, accompanied by a rubber ring to prevent the blood from returning.

VASECTOMY: Sterilization by cutting a part of the vas deferens.

WATCHFUL WAITING: A method of observing prostate cancer, in which treatment is deferred until the disease shows signs of progression.

ZOLADEX: (Zeneca Pharmaceuticals) Synthetic LHRH, used in the treatment of advanced cancer of the prostate.

Prostate Cancer Support Groups

There are several organizations which can offer help to patients with prostate cancer which may vary such as: supplying literature about the cancer and its treatment, or organizing meetings to meet people who have lived through the treatment of this condition. Some organizations may help in finding transportation to the hospitals, doctors, or other treatment centers.

M.D. Anderson
Meets 4th Wed/month
Houston, TX
(713) 792-6195

Man Only/1st Wed/month
St. Martin Episcopal
717 Sage Road
Houston, TX
(713) 792-2553

Meets 2nd Mon/month
St. Lukes Methodist
3417 Westheimer
Houston, TX

Man to Man Support Group
Diagnostic Center
2300 Greek Oaks
Kingwood, TX
(713) 540-7905

US TOO
Jim Charles (713)722-0208
Vernon Witliff
 (713)541-4645

US-TOO
Hinsdale, IL 60521-2993
(708) 323-1002

50+ @ Most Local Hospitals
Prostate Cancer Support
300 W. Pratt St, Suite 401
Baltimore, MD 21201

Patient Advocate for Advanced Cancer (PAACT)
P.O. Box 141695
Grand Rapids, MI 49514
(616) 453-1477

Cancer Care, Inc.
1180 Ave of the Americas
New York, NY 10036
(212) 221-3300

Main Office:
American Cancer Society
1599 Clifton Road NE
Atlanta, GA 30329-4251
1-800-227-2345

Chartered Divisions of The American Cancer Society:

Alaska Division, Inc.
406 W. Fireweed Ln, #204
Anchorage, AK 99503

Alabama Division, Inc.
504 Brookwood Blvd.
Homewood, AL 35209

Arkansas Division, Inc.
901 North University
Little Rock, AR 72207

Arizona Division, Inc.
2929 East Thomas Rd.
Phoenix, AZ 85016

California Division, Inc.
1710 Webster Street
Oakland, CA 94612

Colorado Division, Inc.
2255 South Oneida
Denver, CO 80224

Connecticut Division, Inc.
Barnes Park South
14 Village Lane
Wallingford, CT 06492

District of Columbia Div., Inc.
1875 Conn. Ave., NW, #730
Washington, DC 20009

Delaware Division, Inc.
92 Read's Way
New Castle, DE 19720

Florida Division, Inc.
3709 West Jetton Avenue
Tampa, FL 33629-5146

Georgia Division, Inc.
46 Fifth Street, NE
Atlanta, GA 30308

Hawaii Pacific Division, Inc.
Community Serv. Cntr Bldg.
200 N. Vineyard Blvd #100A
Honolulu, HI 96817

Iowa Division, Inc.
8364 Hickman Road, #D
Des Moines, IA 50325

Idaho Division, Inc.
2676 Vista Avenue
Boise, ID 83705

Illinois Division, Inc.
77 East Monroe
Chicago, IL 60603-5795

Indiana Division, Inc.
8730 Commerce Park Place
Indianapolis, IN 46268

Kansas Division, Inc.
1315 SW Arrowhead Road
Topeka, KS 66604

Kentucky Division, Inc.
701 W. Muhammad Ali Blvd.
Louisville, KY 40201-1807

Louisiana Division, Inc.
837 Gravier Street, #700
New Orleans, LA 70112

Maine Division, Inc.
52 Federal Street
Brunswick, ME 04011

Maryland Division, Inc.
8219 Town Center Drive
Baltimore, MD 21236-0026

Massachusetts Division, Inc.
247 Commonwealth Ave.
Boston, MA 02116

Michigan Division, Inc.
1205 East Saginaw Street
Lansing, MI 48906

Minnesota Division, Inc.
3316 West 66th Street
Minneapolis, MN 55435

Mississippi Division, Inc.
1380 Livingston Lane
Lakeover Office Park
Jackson, MS 39213

Missouri Division, Inc.
3322 American Avenue
Jefferson City, MO 65102

Montana Division, Inc.
17 North 26th
Billings, MT 59101

North Carolina Division, Inc.
11 S. Boylan Avenue, #221
Raleigh, NC 27603

North Dakota Division, Inc.
123 Roberts Street
Fargo, ND 58102

Nebraska Division, Inc.
8502 West Center Road
Omaha, NE 68124-5255

New Hampshire Div, Inc.
Gail Singer Memorial Bldg.
360 Route 101, Unit 501
Bedford, NH 03110-5032

New Jersey Division, Inc.
2600 US Highway 1
North Brunswick, NJ 08902

New Mexico Division, Inc.
5800 Lomas Blvd., NE
Albuquerque, NM 87110

Nevada Division, Inc.
1325 East Harmon
Las Vegas, NV 89119

New York City Division, Inc.
19 West 56th Street
New York, NY 10019

New York State Div, Inc.
6725 Lyons Street
East Syracuse, NY 13057

Long Island Division, Inc.
75 Davids Drive
Hauppauge, NY 11788

Queens Division, Inc.
11225 Queens Boulevard
Forest Hills, NY 11375

Westchester Division, Inc.
30 Glenn Street
White Plains, NY 10603

Ohio Division, Inc.
5555 Frantz Road
Dublin, OH 43017

Oklahoma Division, Inc.
3000 United Founders Blvd.,
#136
Oklahoma City, OK 73112

Oregon Division, Inc.
0330 SW Curry
Portland, OR 97201

Pennsylvania Division, Inc.
Route 422 & Sipe Avenue
Hershey, PA 17033-0897

Philadelphia Division, Inc.
1422 Chestnut Street
Philadelphia, PA 19102

Puerto Rico Division, Inc.
Calle Alverio #577
Esquina Sargento Medina
Hato Rey, PR 00918

Rhode Island Division, Inc.
400 Main Street
Pawtucket, RI 02860

South Carolina Division, Inc.
128 Stonemark Ln.
Westpark Plaza
Columbia, SC 29210

South Dakota Division, Inc.
4101 Carnegie Place
Sioux Falls, SD 57106-2322

Tennessee Division, Inc.
1315 Eighth Avenue South
Nashville, TN 37203

Texas Division, Inc.
2433 Ridgepoint Drive
Austin, TX 78754

Utah Division, Inc.
941 East 3300 South
Salt Lake City, UT 84106

Vermont Division, Inc.
13 Loomis Street
Montpelier, VT 05602

Virginia Division, Inc.
4240 Park Place Court
Glen Allen, VA 23060

Washington Division, Inc.
2120 First Avenue North
Seattle, WA 98109-1140

Wisconsin Division, Inc.
615 North Sherman Avenue
Madison, WI 53704

West Virginia Division, Inc.
2428 Kanawha Blvd, East
Charleston, WV 25311

Wyoming Division, Inc.
2222 Houst Avenue
Cheyenne, WY 82001

ABOUT THE AUTHOR

Dr. Ayaz M. Durrani, is a board certified urologist and a clinical instructor in urology at the University of Texas Health Science Center Houston. He is a staff urologist at the Memorial Hospital Southwest Houston.

Dr. Durrani, received his postgraduate training in surgery for 9 years in England. He is a fellow of the Royal College of Surgeons. In the U.S., he completed his training in urology in 1976 at the Lahey Clinic Foundation, Boston, Mass.

Since then he has been in private practice of urology. Dr. Durrani lectures and writes on the subject of prostate cancer and has developed an instrument which is being used in prostate surgery at several places in the country.

OTHER BOOKS BY SWAN PUBLISHING

HOW NOT TO BE LONELY—If you're about to marry, recently divorced or widowed, want to forgive, forget or both, this is an excellent book; candid, positive, entertaining and informative—answers that will help you get a date or a mate. Over 3 million copies sold . . . . $ 9.95

NEW FATHER'S BABY GUIDE—Another best selling book by Pete Billac. The **perfect gift** for ALL new fathers. There is not a book for new fathers quite like this one! Tells about Lamaze, burping, feeding and changing the baby plus 40 side-splitting cartoons. Most of all how to **SPOIL** mom! GET IT for Dad! . . . . $ 9.95

HOW TO BUY A NEW CAR & SAVE THOU$ANDS—Never be a new car buyer victim again! Inside information on dealerships and sales techniques. Cliff Evans, veteran salesman, gives you inside tips on negotiating, trade-ins, and scams. Really will save you *thousands* on your next car purchase . . . . $ 9.95

REVERSING IMPOTENCE *FOREVER*—A truly great book written by two world famous urologists, Dr. David F. Mobley and Dr. Steven K. Wilson. This books tells MEN how they can REVERSE this problem complete with many drawings which show how impotence can be reversed . . . . $ 9.95

ALL ABOUT CRUISES—Shirley Ragusa (cruise expert) and Pete Billac (63 cruises) tells everything first-time cruisers need to know, about which cruise ships to take, the best deals, shopping, packing, tours, etc. **The best cruise book available!** . . . . $ 9.95

THE TRUTH ABOUT VASECTOMY AND REVERSAL— Facts about frequently asked questions, costs, procedures, explanations on the male reproductive system, contraceptives, patient options and reversals detailed in everyday terms by one of the countries leading urologists, Dr. A.M. Durrani. Complete with photos and glossary of terms . . . . $ 9.95

ALL ABOUT TREES IN & AROUND HOUSTON—Tree expert, John Foster, tells everything you need to know about selecting the best trees, planting, pruning, fertilizing, diagnosing diseases, root barriers & more . . . . $ 9.95

GOLFER'S GUIDE TO GARDENING—Quick, easy methods for gardeners who want a beautiful garden with the least effort and expense. Tips for planting annuals, shrubs, trees; the latest on soils, mulches, insecticides, care for lawns & flower beds by KTRH GardenLine's Randy Lemmon . . . . $ 9.95

BOOKS BY TOM TYNAN:

Volume 1. Home Improvement *Homeowner's most often asked questions*—Saves you thousands of dollars on easy-to repair items in your home that **you** can do! . . . . $ 9.95

Volume 2. Building and Remodeling—How to setup for a large job. Whether you should do it or have it done. How to choose a contractor, subs, get a loan, call an inspection, get permits, insurance, architects, etc. . . . . $ 9.95

Volume 3. Buying & Selling A Home—A book used by many Realtors. Secrets on selling and on buying. What to fix and, what **not** to fix. What to paint. What to clean. Where to get the greatest return on your dollar. A **great** book! . . . . $ 9.95

Volume 4. Step by Step 15 Energy-Saving Projects—Simple, inexpensive projects for your home that will save you money on your energy bills . . . . $ 9.95

BOOKS BY JOHN BURROW:

Your Front Yard—Everything you need to know about growing healthy grass, shrubs and flowers. Answers most homeowners are afraid to ask. A quick reference guide . . . . $ 9.95

Vegetable Gardening *Spring & Fall*—What to grow and when to grow it; in city, country, even patio gardens. Vegetables from A to Z. The vegetable book planting guide for Texas . . $ 9.95

Dr. Durrani has two office locations:

Southwest Memorial Hospital Professional Bldg.
7777 Southwest Freeway, Suite 1068
Houston, TX 77074
713-776-1157

Angleton Danbury Hospital Professional Building
146 Hospital Drive
Angleton, TX 77515
409-849-1201

Dr. A.M. DURRANI is available for personal appearances, luncheons, banquets, seminars, etc.
Call (281) 388-2547 for cost and availability.

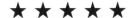

For each book, send a personal check or money order in the amount of $12.85 per copy to:

Swan Publishing
126 Live Oak
Alvin, TX, 77511

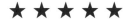

LIBRARIES—BOOKSTORES—QUANTITY ORDERS

To order by major credit card 24 hours a day call:
(713) 268-6776 or long distance 1-800-866-8962
Fax: (281) 585-3738

Delivery in 2-7 days